UN-COMMON SENSE

A PRACTICAL GUIDE FOR HEALTH, WEIGHT LOSS & VITALITY

INCLUDES A 12 WEEK 'INCH LOSS' PROGRAMME

Enjoy!

Ollie

OLLIE MARTIN

A CIP catalogue record for this book is available from the British Library.

Design services from Beth Snowden of The Write Factor
www.thewritefactor.co.uk/www.sixeight.co.uk

FOR JULIA

CONTENTS

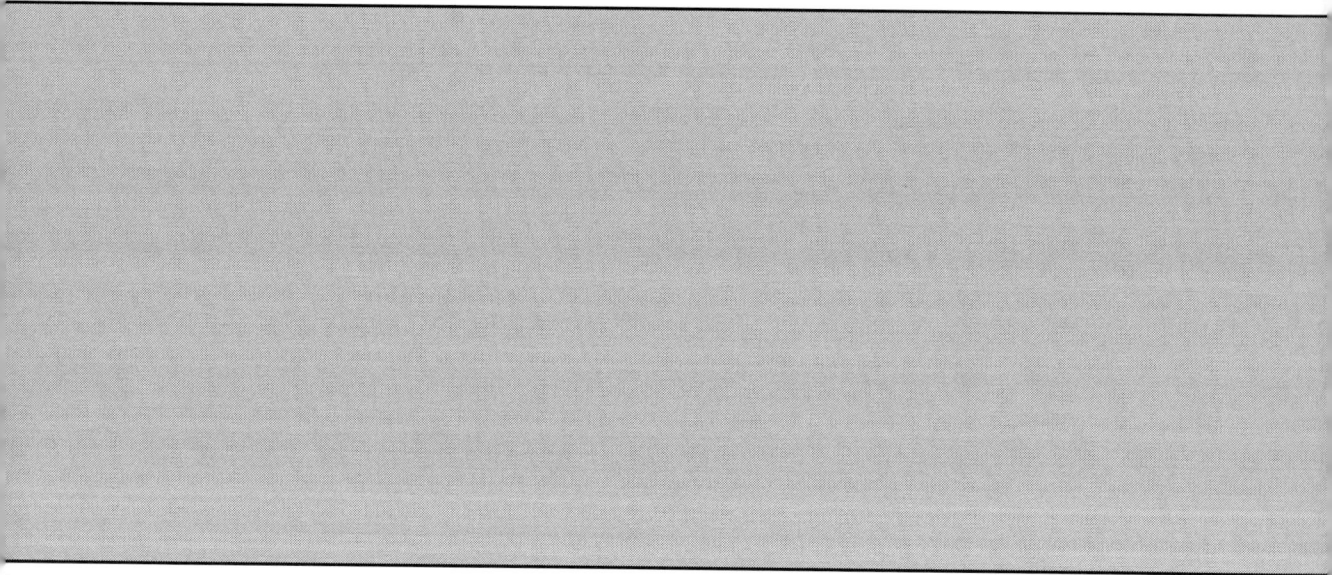

WHAT PEOPLE ARE SAYING ABOUT THE 'UNCOMMON SENSE' APPROACH

"WHAT ABOUT THE FLAT STOMACH? – WELL I LOST 3 INCHES OFF MY WAIST! MY THANKS TO OLLIE MY TRAINER WHO HAS A TREMENDOUS PASSION FOR WHAT HE DOES."

SUE

"EXERCISE COMES EASY TO OLLIE MARTIN. THE FORMER SEMI-PROFESSIONAL RUGBY PLAYER AND OWNER OF TAKE SHAPE IS ONE OF THOSE PEOPLE WHO LOOKS INCREDIBLY FIT, AND DEMONSTRATES EXERCISES FOR YOU TO FOLLOW WITH CONSUMMATE EASE. BUT HE IS ALSO A DRIVEN MAN. DRIVEN TO BE THE BEST AND TO GET THE BEST OUT OF OTHERS. HE PASSIONATELY BELIEVES HE CAN HELP ANYONE IMPROVE THEMSELVES NO MATTER WHAT CONDITION THEY ARE IN FROM YOUNG TO OLD, RECREATIONAL OR PROFESSIONAL ATHLETE."

SURREY MIRROR

"OLLIE'S WIDER EXPERTISE IN HEALTH AND WELLBEING HAS ALLOWED ME TO PROGRESS MY RECOVERY EVEN FURTHER, AND MY ENERGY CONTINUES TO RISE EXPONENTIALLY, EVEN THOUGH I AM RECOVERED BY ANY TRADITIONAL MEASUREMENT. IF I HAD WORKED WITH A CONVENTIONAL TRAINER, I BELIEVE THEY MAY HAVE PUSHED ME BACK INTO ILLNESS. OLLIE UNDERSTANDS THE LINK BETWEEN EXERCISE AND STRESS, AND HOW REST AND RECOVERY IS SO IMPORTANT BOTH IN OUR WORK LIVES, AND IN OUR EXERCISE AND MOVEMENT ACTIVITIES. HE IS ALSO PASSIONATE ABOUT PLAYFUL FUN-BASED MOVEMENT, AND HOW THIS CAN NOT ONLY ENCOURAGE PEOPLE TO MOVE MORE, BUT HOW IT CAN ALSO MAKE MOVEMENT LESS STRESSFUL ON THE NERVOUS SYSTEM."

NICK

"I WAS IN BAD SHAPE. THE TRAINING HAS BEEN MARVELLOUS AND HAS INSPIRED ME TO CONTINUE. THE LOSS OF A DRESS SIZE HAS BEEN THE WINNING FACTOR."

SARAH

"OLLIE HAS HELPED ME KEEP ACTIVE IN MY RETIREMENT AND HAS ENABLED ME TO ENJOY DOING THE THINGS I LOVE. THE TRAINING HAS DEFINITELY IMPROVED MY GOLF AND HAS HELPED ME LOSE A STONE."

LAURIE

"MY WHOLE LIFESTYLE HAS CHANGED, NOT JUST IN TERMS OF FITNESS BUT ALSO IN TERMS OF WEIGHT, SHAPE AND MENTAL TOUGHNESS. IT WOULD BE AN UNDERSTATEMENT TO SAY THAT I FEEL AMAZING. I HAVE LOST LOADS OF WEIGHT AND FEEL GREAT AS A RESULT OF HIS TRAINING, AND I DON'T INTEND TO GO BACK TO THE WAY I WAS BEFORE."

STEPHEN

I'VE LOST FAIR AMOUNT OF WEIGHT AND AM NOW WAKING UP WITH MORE ENERGY AND FEWER ACHES AND PAINS. I HAVE SIGNIFICANTLY MORE ENERGY WHEN PLAYING WITH MY DAUGHTER WHICH IS AN EXERCISE PROGRAMME IN IT'S OWN RIGHT! THE BREATHING/RELAXATION EXERCISES WORK EXTREMELY WELL. I DO THESE EVERY DAY IN THE EVENING AND I DO BELIEVE THESE HAVE ASSISTED GREATLY IN ME SLEEPING BETTER. MY POSTURE IS BETTER AND I HAVE LOST THE TYRE AROUND THE MIDDLE."

MARK

"NOT HAVING BEEN TO A GYM BEFORE BUT, KNOWING I HAD TO ADDRESS MY INCREASING WAISTLINE AND PROBLEMATIC STOMACH (WHICH THE SPECIALIST THOUGHT WAS IBS), I CONTACTED OLLIE FOR A CHAT! BEFORE MEETING OLLIE I DID NOT KNOW WHAT PROGRAMME TO OPT FOR SO, HE TAILOR-MADE ONE FOR ME AND OFF I WENT THINKING I AM GOING TO MAKE THIS WORK FOR ME! AROUND 12 WEEKS LATER, AFTER LISTENING AND TAKING OLLIE'S ADVICE, COMPLETING QUESTIONNAIRES AND STICKING TO A PERSONAL TRAINING / NUTRITION PROGRAMME BUT, NOT DIETING, I HAVE LOST 7 CENTREMETRES FROM MY WAISTLINE. BUT, MOST IMPORTANTLY I FEEL SO MUCH BETTER WITH MORE ENERGY AND NO STOMACH PAINS! OLLIE HAS A GREAT PASSION FOR WHAT HE DOES AND I CANNOT RECOMMEND HIS ADVICE AND TRAINING MORE!"

DIANE

THE UNCOMMON SENSE

When the Dalai Lama was asked what surprised him most about humanity, he said:

"MAN, BECAUSE HE SACRIFICES HIS HEALTH IN ORDER TO MAKE MONEY. THEN HE SACRIFICES HIS MONEY TO RECUPERATE HIS HEALTH. AND THEN HE IS SO ANXIOUS ABOUT THE FUTURE THAT HE DOESN'T ENJOY THE PRESENT; THE RESULT BEING THAT HE DOES NOT LIVE IN THE PRESENT OR THE FUTURE; HE LIVES AS HE IS NEVER GOING TO DIE AND THEN DIES HAVING NEVER REALLY LIVED."

FOREWORD/CASE STUDY

On my 36th birthday I woke up feeling fluey and tired. My throat was tight and my head felt 'muzzy'. Over the following weeks these symptoms worsened, particularly in the days following exercise or having a couple of drinks. The feelings I experienced were nothing like anything I had ever experienced before. I had batteries of standard medical tests including blood tests and ultrasound scans. Apparently I was in perfect health…except I felt terrible. Ultimately, I was diagnosed with 'post-viral fatigue' and then M.E./C.F.S. (Chronic Fatigue Syndrome).

Little did I know that this was the beginning of eight torturous, often unhappy years. I was never bedbound like so many unfortunate people who suffer with ME/CFS; although there were many days during the eight years of my illness when all I felt like doing was curling up in bed and crying. Life was simply too tiring and too unpleasant; too painful and too limiting. I felt exhausted and sick all the time with the thick 'muzzy' head, sore tight throat and an aching body. I had stomach cramps and loose stools every day for over three years – having up to ten bowel movements by ten o'clock in the morning. I would often feel an unpleasant combination of nausea and light-headedness and a sensation of being on the verge of passing out. I would get stinging headaches with the sensation spreading through my whole body as if someone had poured acid through the top of my head. My head and neck locked up so that turning my head even a fraction would be accompanied by excruciating pain. My mouth and tongue could become so swollen and ulcerated that even eating was painful. These were some of the core everyday symptoms. If I 'overdid it", by which I mean maybe doing more than around 15 minutes gentle walking in the day, or talking for too long, things would get much worse.

All this was made all the more frustrating given where I had come from; I had a successful career and worked hard, I loved sports and spent much of my spare time in the gym, in the pool or on my bike. I was fit, healthy and - in my eyes - almost indestructible.

I never listened to the people who said I could not recover, but spent those eight years researching and experimenting with a myriad of differing health approaches. I looked deeply into nutrition, psychology and my emotional make-up. The many different approaches I embraced included Acupuncture, Alexander Technique, Cranial Osteopathy, Lymphatic Drainage, Kinesiology, Massage, different breathing methodologies, and graded activity. I also spent thousands of pounds on food supplements and adopted numerous different dietary approaches.

As I began to recover my health, I started to look more widely at what it takes to achieve sustainable and vibrant health and performance. I spoke to Ollie when I had improved enough to want to accelerate my physical training; I still had to be careful about 'overdoing it' and wanted to work with someone who could help me build my fitness and health but who had the wider understanding of health that my situation demanded.

As I came to understand more and more about Ollie's approach, I realised that it mirrored almost perfectly the lessons I had learned from 8 hard years of personal exploration and recovery.

Whilst I doubt that many of those reading this book have sunk into the depths of chronic illness that I did, the lessons remain the same. Many of you WILL have sub-optimal adrenal function - or adrenal fatigue — that in itself results in sub-optimal health, energy and performance, but which can also be a precursor to more serious illnesses like Chronic Fatigue Syndrome. In *The Ten Uncommon Senses*, Ollie explains how adrenal fatigue is a symptom of the modern environment and lifestyles, and how you can avoid it, and instead lead a life of sustainable energy, health and optimal performance.

Furthermore, Ollie's methodology — whilst highly researched and the result of years of professional insight — is simple to grasp and to apply in every day life. Working with Ollie allowed me to distil my own thinking, and he opened me up to new areas that flowed naturally from my existing understanding, and made absolute intuitive sense.

We live in an age where there has never been more information about health and fitness available to the public. Why then do we also live in a world of escalating obesity, diabetes, cancer, heart disease and general ill health? There are a number of often-interconnected reasons, but these include:

1   Conventional wisdom which is sometimes flawed or misconstrued

2   A lack of motivation to follow a healthy lifestyle

Ollie's approach cuts through these issues. His 'primal-lens' provides the reader with a simple tool to establish what is healthy and what is not (it's tough to argue with millions of years of evolution!). His fun, play based approach to movement and life itself ensures that exercise will no longer feel like a bore, but an opportunity to squeeze the juice from life until the pips squeak!

I hope you enjoy Ollie's book. What is certain, is that if you start to follow the ideas inside then you'll open yourself up to more enjoyment, better health, and enhanced performance at work, to name but a few of the many benefits.

I wish I had discovered these life secrets earlier, but I am so grateful that I know them now.

NICK THOMAS

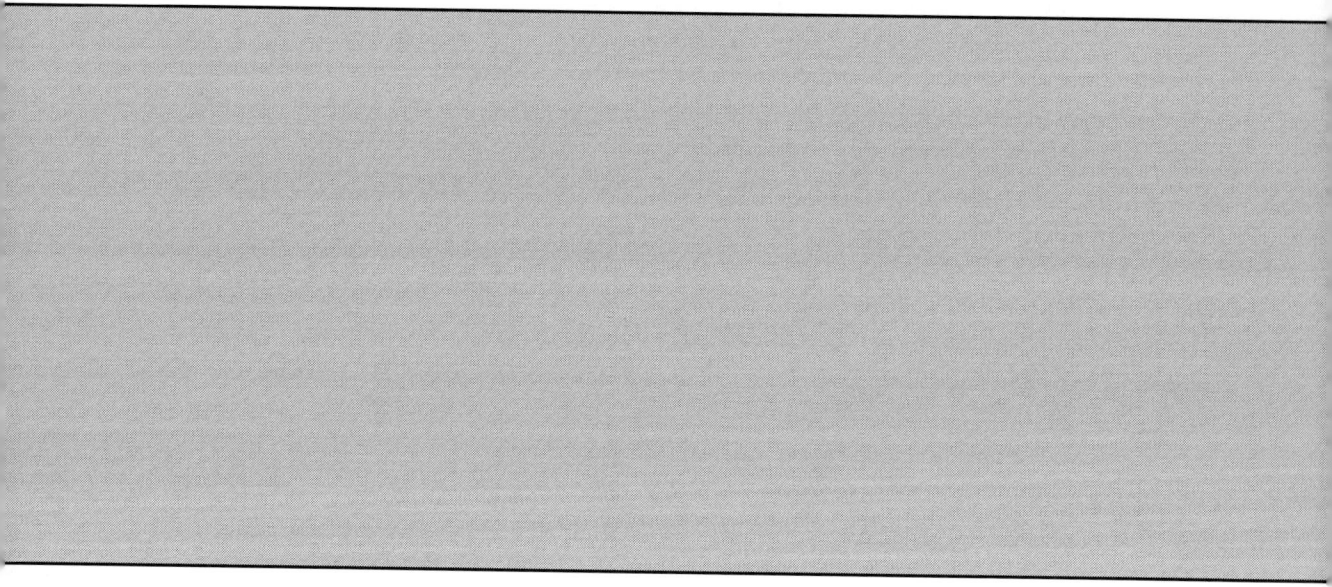

INTRODUCTION

A PRACTICAL GUIDE

The information in this book was initially written as a manual for my clients to help them achieve the best possible results. It gave them a full understanding of what was needed and explained why the coaching was sometimes unconventional! I have now made this available in book form, so that others can get the same results and have fun in doing so.

Each chapter or *Uncommon Sense* (UCS) #1-10 is structured in the sections below:

- At a Glance
- The Paleo Lens
- Some Detail
- Practical Implementation

The approach is intended to be practical and user-friendly; the sections 'At a Glance' and 'Practical Implementation' provide the core information you need to know. Additional detail is provided for those who wish to dig a little deeper.

UNCOMMON SENSE

So what do I mean when I talk about Uncommon Sense?

"A PROBLEM CANNOT BE SOLVED ON THE SAME LEVEL AS CREATED IT"
EINSTEIN

This book might contradict what you know but, a little uncommon sense is needed when we see what a conventional approach has achieved:

- I billion adults in the world are overweight
- 300 million are obese (one in four Adults)
- Nine in 10 will be overweight or obese by 2050
- 121 million people in worldwide are chronically depressed (one in 10 adults)
- One out of every 13 Europeans is currently taking an SSRI (selective serotonin reuptake inhibitor) antidepressant such as Prozac to 'treat' Depression
- There was little or no chronic heart disease before 1920, whereas it is now the number 1 cause of death
- Escalating Risk of Cancer (2nd highest cause of death)
  1900 – 1 person in 30
  1980 – 1 person in 5
  1990 – 1 person in 4
  1995 – 1 person in 3
  2000 – 1 person in 2
- Doctors and medical interventions are the number 3 highest cause of death!

"But, we're living longer…" I hear you protest!

Yes, strictly this is true, but are we truly 'living'? Does spending billions of dollars and pounds keeping people alive but in poor health really constitute 'living' life?

Whilst I leave you to chew on that, consider also that primitive cultures have been shown to live to one hundred years old without 'medical help'. For example, The Journal of the American Medical Association (1961) reported that in the Hunza region, a remote area in the Himalayan Mountains, healthy people lived to be 120 or even 140 years of age.

WHERE WE CAME FROM...THE PALEO LENS

"WHEN WE TRY TO PICK OUT ANYTHING BY ITSELF, WE FIND IT HITCHED TO EVERYTHING ELSE IN THE UNIVERSE."

JOHN MUIR

Many scientific studies examine the body in isolation as if it just landed here from outer space and ignoring 4 million years of evolution.

I believe a more appropriate methodology is to view life through a **'paleo lens'**; in essence, this means that we should evaluate every bit of information according to whether it would make evolutionary sense. Each one of the *Ten Uncommon Senses* includes a section on the paleo lens, which examines the *Uncommon Sense* in an evolutionary context to explain why it will help you.

LOOKING THROUGH A 'PALEO LENS' WILL SHOW YOU WHY THE 'UNCOMMON SENSE' WILL HELP YOU ACHIEVE YOUR DESIRED RESULTS

WHERE WE ARE NOW...

You might think that some of the suggestions in this book are unconventional, unscientific or unknown. But, be careful what you dismiss…

"THE BIGGEST SCIENTIFIC DELUSION OF ALL IS THAT SCIENCE ALREADY KNOWS THE ANSWERS."

RUPERT SHELDRAKE

The irony of science is that people quote it with evangelical certainty. If that were the case there would be no need for continued science! Scientists are the first to admit that the world is full of unsolved mysteries, the ongoing applications for millions of pounds of research grants and the current Large Hadron Collider project would attest to that. *The universe is not a done deal, science is a work in progress.*

The leading thinkers of their day thought the world was flat.

Galileo Galilei, 'the father of modern science', was ridiculed, put under house arrest and accused of heresy in the 1600's for suggesting that the earth revolved around sun (he was forgiven by the Pope 300 years later!).

In 1800's Dr Ignaz Semmelweis, an early pioneer of anti-sceptic procedures, was ostracised by his fellow doctors because they didn't want to wash their hands. Semmelweis's findings earned widespread acceptance only years after his death, when Louis Pasteur confirmed the germ theory.

"WHAT IS NOW PROVED WAS ONCE ONLY IMAGINED."

WILLIAM BLAKE

So please consider the suggestions in this book with an open-mind. When you view them through the paleo lens, I think you will begin to notice that they make intuitive sense. When you try them out for yourself, I know that your body and mind will feel the difference, and the results will prove it!

HEALTH, DISEASE AND WEIGHT LOSS

Before charging headlong into considering the *Uncommon Senses*, it is important to provide some context around what supports health and creates disease, and about where weight loss fits into this equation.

Generally, my clients come to see me to improve their performance in a certain area of their life, but 'weight loss' is often at least a secondary goal. My first task is to help my client understand that weight loss is not something that can be treated in isolation. This is a difficult one because all the information clients have been 'fed' up to this point - from diet companies, doctors, media, and food manufacturers – have centred on the principle of an isolated, instant fix to achieve weight loss and bikini-model style mid-riffs!

Health and weight loss are inextricably linked. Being overweight is a sign that your body is out of balance; it is a small but significant early warning that your health is being compromised in some way. Medical research is also correlating being overweight, and especially being obese, with disease.

So yes, weight and percentage bodyfat, and the distribution of that bodyfat is important. But, I hope that by the time you have read this book, you will understand why a focus on weight loss will never lead to long-term weight optimisation and happiness with the way you look. Instead, you will understand that a focus on real health, through the *Ten Uncommon Senses*, will free you from 'yo-yo dieting' and give you the body you want. You will also enjoy improved skin, greater energy and vitality, a strong core and back, and optimal performance in everything you do. *Is that all?* No, but, it's enough to be getting with!

HEALTH AND THE ADRENALS

Tired for no reason?
Having trouble getting up in the morning?
Need coffee, carbonated drinks, salty or sweet snacks to keep going?
Feeling run down and stressed?
Have difficulty in losing weight?

If you answered yes to one or more of these questions, you are experiencing adrenal fatigue. It is estimated that as many as 90% of adults in this country have some degree of adrenal fatigue!

Adrenal fatigue can affect anyone who experiences frequent, persistent or severe mental, emotional or physical stress. It can also be an important contributing factor in health conditions ranging from allergies to obesity. Despite its prevalence in our modern world, adrenal fatigue has generally been ignored and misunderstood by the medical community.

WHAT CAUSES ADRENAL FATIGUE?

Adrenal fatigue is produced when your adrenal glands cannot adequately meet the demands of stress. The adrenal glands mobilise your body's responses to every kind of stress (whether it's physical, emotional, or psychological) through hormones that regulate energy production and storage, immune function, heart rate, muscle tone, and other processes that enable you to cope with the stress. Whether you experience an emotional crisis such as the death of a loved one, a physical crisis such as major surgery, or any type of severe repeated or constant stress in your life, your adrenals have to respond to the stress and maintain health. If their response is inadequate, you are likely to experience some degree of adrenal fatigue.

During adrenal fatigue your adrenal glands function, but not well enough to maintain optimal homeostasis, because their output of regulatory hormones has been diminished - usually by over-stimulation. Over-stimulation of your adrenals can be caused either by a very intense single stress, or by chronic or repeated stresses that have a cumulative effect.

"STRESS IS THE UNDERLYING CAUSE OF ALL ILLNESS"

DR MICHAEL KUCERA

BALANCE OF STRESSORS

"A STRESSOR IS ANYTHING IN THE OUTSIDE WORLD THAT KNOCKS YOU OUT OF HOMEOSTATIC BALANCE, AND THE STRESS RESPONSE IS WHAT YOUR BODY DOES TO RE-ESTABLISH HOMEOSTASIS."

SAPOLSKY

The word stress is much discussed and even more misunderstood! Stress is normally seen as bad, but stress is neither bad nor good. Only the consequences of the 'balance of stressors', one way or another, can be good or bad. For example, exercise is a stressor as it tears individual muscle tissues, but it is beneficial because it stimulates repair and subsequent super-compensation. This results in fitter and stronger muscle tissue for use next time it is called upon.

Our bodies are designed through evolution to deal with short, sharp stressors such as a predator (e.g. sabre-tooth tiger) attack. This major stressor will stimulate our fight/flight response, where we either fight this tiger off or run away. In such a situation we will either be eaten or get away. If we get away, the stress was a short, sharp, acute stressor, which completely disappears as quickly as it came…and if we don't get away, then we would be dead anyway! However, today's stressors are more long-term, low level, chronic stressors such as mortgages, jobs, pollution etc. These affect our primal bodies adversely by continually suppressing our rest and repair.

AUTONOMIC NERVOUS SYSTEM

The automonic nervous system controls the body's stress response. You are either using your Sympathetic Nervous System (SNS) which is your "Fight/Flight" mode. Or you are in your Parasympathetic Nervous System (PNS) which is your "Rest & Repair" mode. Balance is needed between the two, a dominance in one or other will causes dis-harmony and dis-ease. In 21st Century living most people are too sympathetically dominant until 'adrenal fatigue' sets in and they become too parasympathetically dominant.

FUNCTIONAL RESERVE

Stress can be physical, chemical, emotional, mental or geothermal, but it is treated by the body in the same way, and depletes the same 'functional reserve' pot:

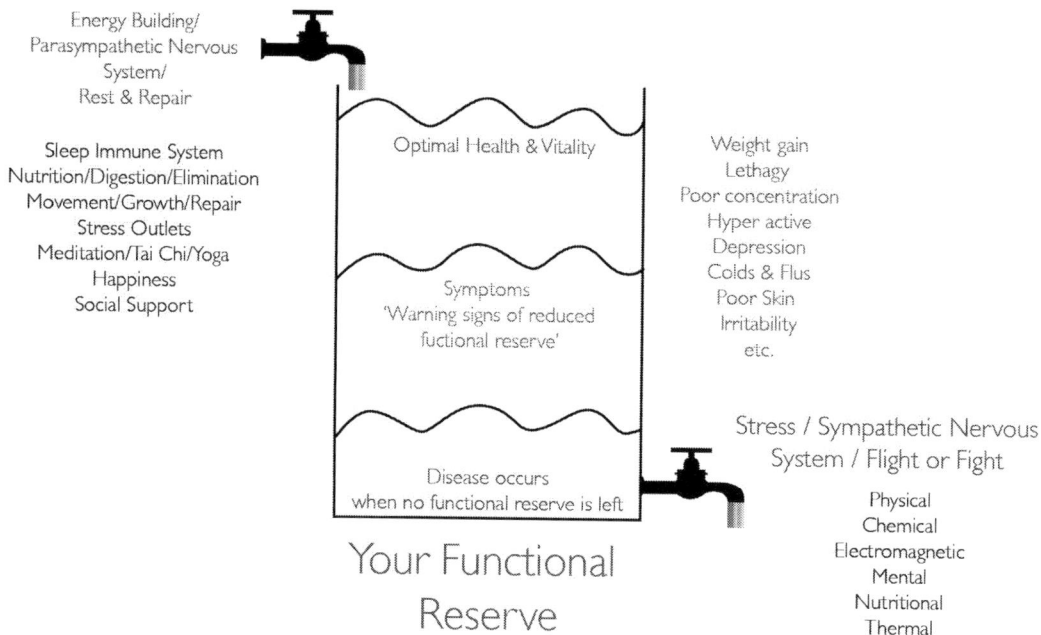

Energy Building/
Parasympathetic Nervous
System/
Rest & Repair

Sleep Immune System
Nutrition/Digestion/Elimination
Movement/Growth/Repair
Stress Outlets
Meditation/Tai Chi/Yoga
Happiness
Social Support

Optimal Health & Vitality

Symptoms
'Warning signs of reduced
fuctional reserve'

Disease occurs
when no functional reserve is left

Weight gain
Lethagy
Poor concentration
Hyper active
Depression
Colds & Flus
Poor Skin
Irritability
etc.

Stress / Sympathetic Nervous
System / Flight or Fight

Physical
Chemical
Electromagnetic
Mental
Nutritional
Thermal

Your Functional
Reserve

Functional Reserve is the body's bank account. If you spend more than you save, you will deplete your functional reserve.

The body has a 'functional reserve' to deal with any problems arising in the body. When this reserve is depleted the body has nothing to combat these problems and disease will set in. So, if an individual has an illness or disease, it is not the illness or disease that has caused the problem, it is the depleted functional reserve.

Younger people generally have fewer problems fighting off disease and recovering from injury because they have ample functional reserves. As one gets older and the functional reserve is depleted, there is nothing left to combat stressors. This leads to poor performance, illness, injury and disease. It is also why a perceived small stressor can cause a huge health problem; this is the proverbial 'straw that breaks the camel's back'!

Therefore, to remain healthy the body must look after its functional reserve, and through doing so, it ages less quickly, looking and performing better.

STATE-OF-THE-ART FUNCTIONAL RESERVE WARNING SYSTEM – A STANDARD FEATURE ON ALL MODELS

All humans possess a state-of-the-art monitoring system as a standard feature to let them know when the functional reserve is being compromised. This monitoring system issues warning signs, which we often refer to as 'symptoms'!

DID YOU KNOW A HEADACHE IS NOT AN ASPIRIN DEFICIENCY?

Illness and injury are symptoms and should be welcomed as knowledge and insight into what is happening to an individual's body. However, the current medical paradigm tends to treat these symptoms in isolation and, rather than learning from them, covers them up. This is a missed opportunity for an individual to change their lifestyle accordingly. In particular, lifestyle should be adapted to reduce stress load, preserve functional reserve and combat disease. This gives the individual the energy for optimal performance.

A few signs of reduced functional reserve are: regular colds and infections, lethargy, weight gain, skin problems, fatigue, hyperactivity, illness when going on holiday, restlessness, sleep problems, waking up in the middle of the night, injury, disease, poor concentration, irritability and reliance on stimulants.

IF YOU EXPERIENCE ANY OF THESE SYMPTOMS, TAKE ACTION WITH THE HELP OF THE TEN UNCOMMON SENSES, NOW!

UCS #1:
HIT OR NEAT

AT A GLANCE

HIT – HIGH INTENSITY TRAINING

This is exactly what it says on the tin! The idea is to train very hard for shorts burst of time. Think interval training in the gym, but also sprinting for the bus and some sports scenarios.

NEAT – NON-EXERCISE ACTIVITY THERMOGENESIS

NEAT could be described as any movement that does not get you out of breath; walking, taking the stairs, gardening and housework all qualify!

The best health and weight loss results are achieved by working at these two intensities and not in-between.

HIT = circa 90% MHR (Maximum Heart Rate), circa 9 on a 1-10 RPE scale (Rate of Perceived Exertion – a very good, accurate and easy measure of intensity).

NEAT = circa 50% MHR, circa 5 RPE.

Do not train at the intensity most people train at i.e. 60-85% of MHR because of the stress response and subsequent fat storage.

(See UCS #7)

THE PALEO LENS

Without movement there is no life. Movement = life.

HIT and NEAT are the two intensities that injure the body the least, meaning that the body will recover quicker. NEAT because of the lack of force, impact and technique offsetting (using the wrong muscles to achieve the movement) required. HIT because of the short duration that you can sustain it.

Our ancestors spent a lot of time moving at about 50% of their maximum heart rate, interspersed with very high intensity short bursts. The persistence hunt is a good example of this. As 'hunters' and 'gatherers' we were not blessed with the speed or even strength of our prey such as an antelope; however, we did have some unique 'persistence' abilities that enabled us to track an animal until it died of exhaustion. This is now understood to be one of the main ways that we 'hunted'.

These persistence abilities include:

- The ability to sweat to cool down
- The ability to carry water

Humankind spent millions of years of evolution operating at these intensities; it makes sense that to keep healthy we should replicate what our bodies have been designed for.

SOME DETAIL

The human heart pumps 7200 litres per day everyday day throughout our lives. It is no bigger than a fist and does not get an annual service! To enable smooth running, the heart does need body movement to help it pump blood around the body and back to the heart for oxygenation. Through vasoconstriction - the squeezing of the vessels/arteries - and the valve system, blood is pumped back to the heart. Movement is vital for vasoconstriction.

But, it does not have to be hard to get the results one is looking for. The old school mentality of 'no pain, no gain', and working to the point of exhaustion has too many negatives – injury and the fact it is just plain unpleasant - for it to be beneficial.

Research at Nottingham University found that HIT sessions recorded a 30 percent improvement in the effectiveness in insulin action: that's the body's ability to move glucose out of the bloodstream — 'where it can become a toxin and lead to the build-up of dangerous visceral fat' — and into muscle tissue, where it is of benefit.

PROFESSOR JAMES TIMMONS:

"THE SCIENCE IS DEVELOPING ON HIGH-INTENSITY INTERVAL TRAINING. YES, IT IS REALLY GOOD AT IMPROVING GLUCOSE UPTAKE INTO THE MUSCLES IN A VERY, VERY SHORT TIME. WITH REALLY INTENSE EXERCISE, YOU RELEASE HORMONES THAT CAN HELP BREAK DOWN FAT. THIS MAY HELP BURN THAT FAT OVER TIME, AFTER HIT IS DONE. ALSO, WE THINK, BUT DON'T KNOW, THAT HIT WILL SUBDUE APPETITE, WHILE TRADITIONAL EXERCISE (JOGGING ETC) WILL STIMULATE APPETITE. THIS LAST POINT IS KEY AND WILL BE RESEARCHED BY OUR TEAM."

MARTIN GIBALA, MCMASTER UNIVERSITY IN ONTARIO, CANADA,

"A GROWING BODY OF EVIDENCE DEMONSTRATES THAT HIT CAN SERVE AS AN EFFECTIVE ALTERNATE TO TRADITIONAL ENDURANCE-BASED TRAINING, INDUCING SIMILAR OR EVEN SUPERIOR PHYSIOLOGICAL ADAPTATIONS. SUCH FINDINGS ARE IMPORTANT GIVEN THAT 'LACK OF TIME' REMAINS THE MOST COMMONLY CITED BARRIER TO REGULAR EXERCISE PARTICIPATION."

Most people work just below their anaerobic threshold, at about 7 out of 8 on a scale of perceived exertion. What is wrong with this?

- The paleo lens shows us that it is not in line with our evolutionary heritage, and as a result is inefficient and stressful to our bodies
- Efficiency is comprised by postural compensations due to fatigue
- It is unpleasant to exercise in this way, so not exactly a motivating factor to get people moving!
- Just think how the body perceives this movement. Running fast is seen as the evolutionary mechanism to escape a life-threatening predator. This is fine for short periods of time (see HIT) as the body has time to rest and recover. Moving at this intensity for long periods is highly stressful and depletes functional reserve. Chronic stimulation of the adrenals can lead to adrenal fatigue.

THE KEY TO NEAT IS NOSE BREATHING

We are obligate nose breathers, which means we do not possess the voluntary ability to breath through the mouth. Mouth breathing is a learned response triggered by emergency stress. Look at the breathing of a baby and we see breathing through the nose with the tummy rising on inhalation. Nose breathing allows for deep calm breathing, whereas mouth breathing is shallow and only intended for times of stress. However, through repeated and chronic - long-term – stressors, most of us have developed an inverted breathing pattern where we predominantly breathe through our mouth, and shallow breathe with our tummy coming in rather than out when we inhale. This creates a 'vicious circle', which heightens our stress response.

By nose breathing we have to keep our intensity at about 50 per cent of maximum heart rate. This has the following beneficial effects:

- Lessens stress on the body
- Reduces adrenal response
- Aids quicker recovery
- Maintains posture and efficiency
- Reduces chance of injury

So, to tie in our running training with a 'primal lifestyle' it makes sense to either embark on long, low-intensity outings involving a mix of walking, slow running, climbing, load-bearing (our ancestors will have had to walk long distances carrying their infants, for example); or to practise a wide variety of sprints of various distances and intensities, up to a maximum of around 400m or circa 50 seconds, whichever comes first. Hint – it is circa 50 seconds for majority of us!

SAID PRINCIPLE

The key to getting fit comes down to what we are trying to get fit for, and the SAID Principle – Specific Adaptations to Imposed Demand. In other words, we get what we train for!

If we are training for a 10k run, how do we implement the HIT & NEAT philosophy?

10k is neither a sprint nor very low intensity exercise! In the race, in order to get the best time, we want to run as fast as we can for about an hour. This will be at our anaerobic threshold of about 80% of maximum heart rate. According to the SAID principle we should therefore train at 80% maximum heart rate. However, consider the following points:

- Running a 10k as fast as we can is not an intensity or distance that is in line with our evolutionary heritage, and is therefore the most stressful.
- That doesn't mean we should not do it though because it has many advantages for health such as motivation, enjoyment, achievement, moving body, and getting outside
- But there is a high risk of injury and we will not necessarily achieve the health or weight loss results we want
- The answer is to follow HIT & NEAT training for 90% of the time which will help optimise health and weight, whilst carrying out 10k training for 10% of the time for SAID and performance in our 10k run
- There is a crossover of endurance benefits when HIT training but little the other way

IMPLEMENTATION

BECOME AN EXERCISE OPPORTUNIST - find any opportunity in your day to build gentle movement into your day. Ideally, also build in a short burst of intense exercise. Play is one of the best ways to do this, but more on this later.

HIT IDEAS:

- Interval training e.g. 15 second bursts with 60 seconds rest. Stop when you lose quality/ technique or when the rest period is not enough e.g. when you find you have to rest your hands onto your knees during the recovery period.
- Playing 'IT' with the kids
- Racing the dog
- Power training in the gym e.g. kettlebells, dumbbells, and medicine balls
- Strength training

NEAT IDEAS:

- Build up to 10,000 steps a day (buy a pedometer)
- Use minimalist shoes (more on this in the next chapter)
- Build more movement into every day tasks. For example, take the stairs instead of the lift, and park further from the shops!
- Take your dog for a walk even if you don't have one!
- Take up a sport, dance class, Tai chi, yoga or similar activity
- Engage in a daily evening stretching programme
- 100's more ideas, so do whatever you like that involves moving...

UCS #2:
LESS IS MORE...
FOOTWISE

AT A GLANCE

It may seem counter-intuitive, but exercising/moving (including running) barefoot is more efficient and puts less impact through the body than wearing shoes or trainers.

Barefoot exercise brings the following benefits:

- Reduced impact & injury
- Improved performance
- Better health

PALEO LENS

This is an easy one – we were not born with Nikes on! Trainers have only been around for around 40 years but we have been designed, through evolution, to move great distances without injuring ourselves.

Trainers change our running/moving technique to an unnatural gait that causes injury and reduces performance.

DANIEL LIEBERMAN, HARVARD UNIVERSITY 2012

"HEEL STRIKERS ARE TWICE AS LIKELY TO GET INJURED THAN THOSE THAT DON'T HEEL STRIKE." (NOTE: THE BAREFOOT RUNNING TECHNIQUE IS ALL ABOUT FOREFOOT STRIKING)

STANFORD UNIVERSITY HEAD TRACK COACH VIN LANANNA (APRIL 2001) TO NIKE REPRESENTATIVES:

"...I BELIEVE WHEN MY RUNNERS TRAIN BAREFOOT, THEY RUN FASTER AND SUFFER FEWER INJURIES." WE HAVE SHIELDED OUR FEET FROM THEIR NATURAL POSITION BY PROVIDING MORE AND MORE SUPPORT. STRENGTHEN FEET AND YOU REDUCE THE RISK OF ACHILLES AND PLANTAR FASCIA PROBLEMS.

1989 JOURNAL OF SPORTS MEDICINE

"THE MORE YOU SPEND ON A SHOE THE MORE RISK OF INJURY."

2008 BRITISH JOURNAL OF SPORTS MEDICINE

"THERE ARE NO EVIDENCE-BASED STUDIES (NOT ONE) THAT RUNNING SHOES MAKE YOU LESS PRONE TO INJURY. NO RUNNING SHOE COMPANY WAS PREPARED TO DENY THIS."

SOME DETAIL

But, I hear you say:

I need arch support
I need heel cushioning

In fact, these aspects of modern shoes can be the problem rather than the solution:

If you support something it gets weaker
If you push an arch from below it collapses
If you cushion something it loses sensitivity

The power of modern marketing can distort the truth, and create artificial demand. Many of us now unquestioningly believe that we need these heavily cushioned shoes, whereas in truth, less support and cushioning actually reduce impact on the body. This being said, in recent times there has been some favourable press coverage of the benefits of a more minimalist approach to footwear. This message has reached a wider audience through the cult classic, *Born to Run* by Chris McDougall, which details his amazing travels to the Tarahumara tribe in Mexico.

RESEARCH ON THE BENEFITS OF 'BAREFOOT' RUNNING

- Enhanced running efficiency
- Facilitated venous return resulting in:
  - ▶ Decreased blood pressure
  - ▶ Reduced risk of deep vein thrombosis
  - ▶ Lower incidence of varicose veins

- Decreased ankle sprains
- Lowered risk of shin splints
- Minimize back pain
- Enhanced proprioception
- Strengthens intrinsic foot musculature
- Maximise biomechanical performance
- Diminish risk of bunions
- Optimise balance and prevent falls

Source: Matthew Wallden (www.primalifestyle.com)

'BAREFOOT TED' MACDONALD, ONE OF THE STARS FROM CHRIS MCDOUGAL'S BOOK BORN TO RUN SAYS:

"THE HALLMARK OF MY BAREFOOT RUNNING PHILOSOPHY IS REGAINING CONNECTEDNESS, MINDFULNESS, AND PRESENCE IN YOUR RUNNING AND IN YOUR BODY."

"BAREFOOT RUNNING IS ABOUT TUNING-IN TO YOUR OWN BODY'S HIGHLY SOPHISTICATED SET OF INTEGRATED AWARENESS SYSTEMS, SYSTEMS THAT COMMUNICATE THROUGH FEELINGS AND SENSES THAT ARE BEING COLLECTED IN REAL-TIME AS YOU MOVE. FROM MY PERSPECTIVE, LEARNING HOW TO RUN WELL MEANS LEARNING HOW TO TAP INTO THE FEELING OF RUNNING WELL, WHICH MORE OFTEN THAN NOT REQUIRES BARING THE FOOT TO GET THE FULL FEEL OF WHAT HAPPENS WHEN YOU MOVE."

"PAIN TEACHES YOU HOW TO RUN."

BAREFOOT/EARTHING

We live for extended periods of time completely disconnected from the earth. Today we sleep upstairs and wear man made rubber soles that insulate us further from contact with the earth. With all the dramatic use in electrical equipment, increasing microwave-radiating phone masts, Digital TV and all things wireless (see UCS #8), we are not able to discharge any of the electrical radiation we are being subjected to.

The earth has a negative electrical surface due to the thousands of thunderstorm and lightening strikes every second. Standing barefoot on the earth connects the body with its unlimited supply of health promoting free electrons resident in and on the surface of the earth. This also connects the human body with rhythmic cycles of the earth's energy field, essential for synchronising body clocks, hormonal cycles and physiological rhythms.

PRACTICAL IMPLEMENTATION

"HUMANS ARE OBLIGATORILY REQUIRED TO DO AEROBIC EXERCISE IN ORDER TO STAY HEALTHY, AND I THINK THAT HAS DEEP ROOTS IN OUR EVOLUTIONARY HISTORY,"

"IF THERE'S ANY MAGIC BULLET TO MAKE HUMANS HEALTHY IT IS TO RUN."

DR LEIBERMAN, HARVARD UNIVERSITY

BAREFOOT RUNNING

Barefoot running allows everyone to run injury free, regardless of size, shape or fitness – you are born to run, so recapture your evolutionary heritage.

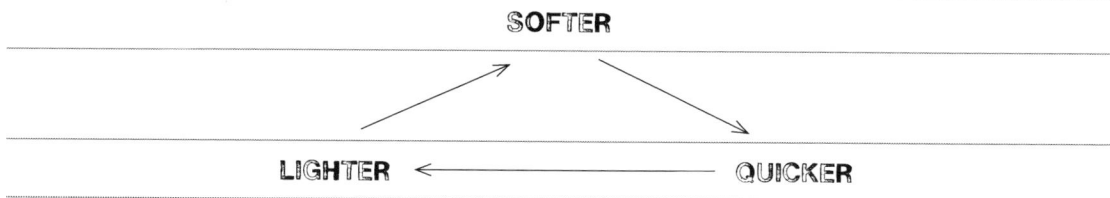

SOFTER

LIGHTER ← QUICKER

SOFTER

- Before you begin, align your posture through a **biomechanical assessment and corrective exercise programme** – this will soften and balance your muscles reducing stress load on your body and eliminate risk of repetitive strain injury
- **Start easy and build up slowly** - a MUST do otherwise you WILL injure yourself
- **Relax** your muscles, sinking shoulders and hips
- **Meditative mindset**: clear your mind, let thoughts that come into your mind drift away without attachment, focus on your breathing and/or the muscles in your body, are they tight? Is there pain? Which ones are working?

- **Train at 50% of your maximum heart rate.** You can do this by keeping to nose, rather than mouth, breathing
- Learn to **listen to your body** – acknowledge and adapt to any pain; barefoot running gives you instant feedback and this is your best teacher

QUICKER

- **Increase foot cadence** - not overall speed…yet. Aim for over 180 foot strikes per minute. Buy a digital metronome or count 1,2,3…
- Your speed will increase with the better efficiency of movement from lower intensities
- Good technique through efficiency will shorten recovery times and reduce risk of injury

LIGHTER

- No pounding the ground - **fluid, silent and smooth**
- You should feel **lightness** through your whole body
- **Forefoot centric foot landing** - the ball of your foot should touch the ground first
- Hard surfaces such as Tarmac are often the best to learn on because of instant feedback
- Use nothing, Vibram Fivefingers or a minimalist shoe – in order of preference. I do not recommend progressive shoes, which reduce support gradually, because you miss the teaching effect of feedback.
- **Enjoy it!**

CONDITIONING/GYM EXERCISES

The following support a barefoot running approach:
- Squat with correct alignment
- Two footed jumping on the spot on the balls of your feet at 180bpm (beats per minute)
- One footed jumping on the spot on the balls of your feet at 180bpm
- Running on the spot at 180bpm
- Skipping at 180bpm

Take your time to condition and learn. This is not an instant fix. If you do not take your time you will injure yourself just as you would in conventional training.

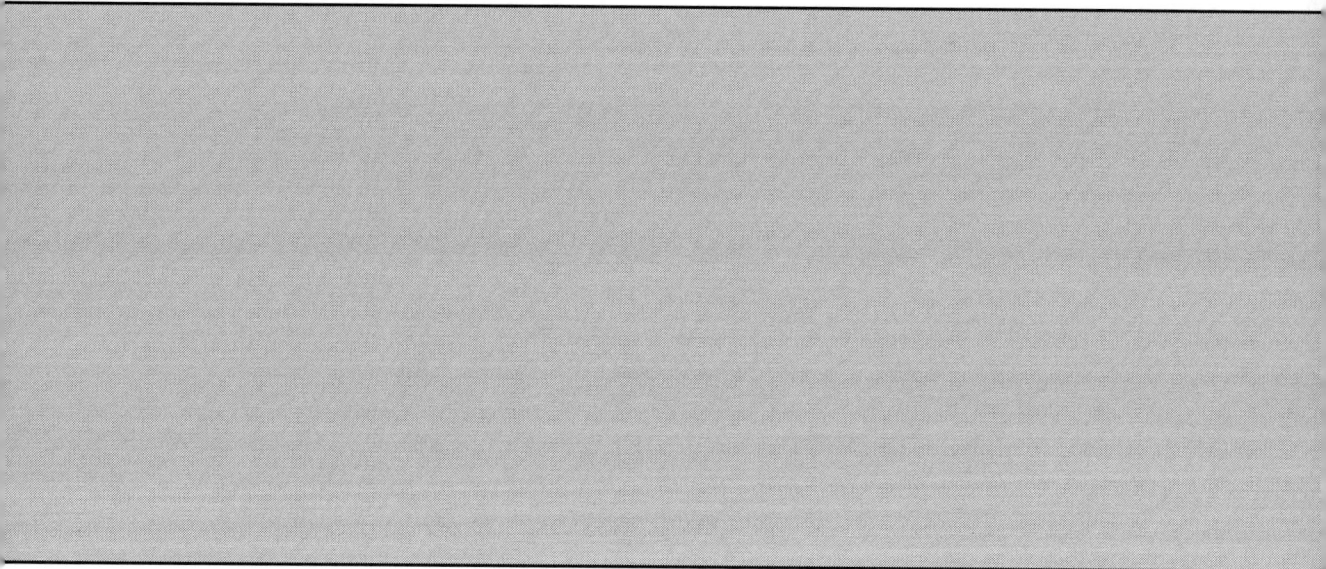

UCS #3:
HAVE FUN

AT A GLANCE

Many people think that being healthy is all about denial, abstinence and the 'no pain, no gain' philosophy. But this is the exact opposite of the truth; fun and playfulness should be at the forefront of your health and weight loss strategy.

IF THE ONLY REASON YOU ARE EXERCISING IS TO GET AN END RESULT, YOU HAVE A POOR CHANCE OF SUCCEEDING. HOWEVER, IF YOUR EXERCISE IS FUN AND YOU ENJOY THE PROCESS, YOU HAVE A VERY HIGH CHANCE OF SUCCEEDING.

Exercise is a wonderful opportunity for you to play, to be creative and to have fun. The simplest point to make is that if you enjoy what you are doing you will do more of it for longer. Ten minutes on a stationary bike in the gym might make you feel self-righteous but it feels like a long time! Kicking a ball around the garden for ten minutes works more muscles, burns more calories and feels like no time at all.

The second point is that that if is not fun it might also be painful and damaging the body. Fun acts as a protection mechanism – the body perceives the movement as less 'stressful'; if you're having fun you know the body will recover well.

IF IT IS NOT FUN, THEN YOU ARE NOT DOING IT RIGHT!

PALEO LENS

PLAY IS KEY TO BEING A HUMAN BEING, AND HOW MUCH YOU PLAY ACTS AS A BAROMETER OF HEALTH

The natural world is ruthless in selecting out individuals with inappropriate physical behaviours. Any young animal that played with inefficient or inappropriate movements would be unlikely to make it to a reproductive age. We can therefore assume that if a movement is fun it will be appropriate for our bodies and consistent with our evolutionary heritage. We can also assume that playful movement patterns are likely to be biomechanically and neurologically correct for our bodies — ideal for long-term, pain free function.

"YOU CAN LEARN MORE ABOUT A PERSON IN AN HOUR OF PLAY THAN A YEAR OF CONVERSATION."

PLATO

SOME DETAIL

FUN IS THE EVOLUTIONARY BASED REWARD FOR LEARNING

NEUROPLASTICITY

In childhood, play is most prevalent in periods of most rapid brain development. This is because play fires up neural connections that do not seem to have an immediate function but are essential to continued brain organisation. In playing we foster creation of new circuits and test them by running signals through them. In adults, unlike animals, we have capacity for new neuron growth well into adulthood, and this growth is stimulated by play.

The human nervous system is incredibly dynamic and constantly re-sculpts itself in response to life experience. The latest science of Epigenics identifies that nurture is more powerful influence than nature on behavior. Not only do we generate new brain cells (neurogenesis), but we also modify connections between cells and insulation around nerve fibres. Collectively, these changes are referred to as neuroplasticity.

So play actually makes us smarter and rewires our circuitry around problems. Unlike computers, the more our circuitry is used, the faster and more efficient the signals between neurons become. This process is called long-term potentiation and is an increasing area of research in neuroscience.

THE MORE YOU PLAY, THE BIGGER YOUR BRAIN

CREATIVITY

Play inspires creativity and innovation by mixing fantasy with reality, the imagination with the 'rules of the game'. Play activates functionally diverse brain regions to synergistically integrate their function resulting in creativity.

SOCIAL COHESION

When people play together, they become attuned to each other.

MENTAL & PHYSICAL HEALTH

Play is not the opposite of work, depression is the opposite of play. Respecting our biologically programmed need for play keeps up mentally and physically fit. Stress is the cause of all illness and laughter is the best antidote to stress.

WE NEED VARIETY AND CHALLENGE

Play brings excitement and adventure back into lives and allows us to fully engage with the world.

MASTERY

To become a master one has to go beyond what can be taught, one needs to play with possibilities, learn from what doesn't work and build on what does work - anything but a playful mindset will lead to frustration and quitting.

FULFILMENT

Play comes from our own inner needs and desires and is the only path to finding lasting joy and satisfaction in our work.

PROBLEM SOLVING

The problem is not the problem, the problem is how you react to the problem. People who have engaged in play throughout their lives and can bring that emotion to their problems are able to do well at work/life related tasks that at first might seem to have no connection to play at all.

"ALWAYS SURPRISE THE BODY"

ARNOLD SCHWARZENEGGER

LEARNING MODEL

The best model for learning I have come across is from David Whitehead. Simplified, this model says you first need to start with romance, to have the student fall in love with the subject. To do this you need to engage the student with the fun aspects of the subject, from which they will receive some immediate joy. Any subject worth learning will then need a disciplined stage, to learn the finer points in order to enable greater proficiency. The third stage is back to romance, the student must fall back in love with the subject to gain mastery.

ROMANCE – DISCIPLINE – ROMANCE...

I use this model for individual movement sessions as well as for ongoing programmes.

PROPERTIES OF PLAY:

- Apparently purposeless - done for its own sake
- Voluntary
- Inherent attraction
- Freedom from time
- Diminished consciousness of self
- Improvisational potential
- Continuation of desire

THE SAID PRINCIPLE VERSUS THE FUN PRINCIPLE

We saw earlier that the body adapts according to the specific demands placed on it (SAID – Specific Adaption to Imposed Demand) which would seem to contradict the idea that 'playing around' will have a positive effect on performance. However, studies have shown that a playful approach to training can achieve a better performance than simply replicating specific movement patterns in training. Hence the benefits of cross-training. For example, a study where participants threw balls into a bucket found that those which 'played around' with the distance away from the bucket achieved better results than those that kept the same distance away from the bucket. Therefore, a blend of SAID and Fun produces the greatest impetus for performance improvement.

PRACTICAL IMPLEMENTATION

PERMISSION

- First of all give yourself permission to be playful. Many think that 'playing around' is a waste of time or childish. I'm telling you it is not but, you also need to tell yourself that it is alright and actually beneficial to make time for play.

FOCUS

- Make having fun be a focus in life. More on this when we talk about values in UCS#10 but, where you direct your attention has a direct reflection on what you get back in terms of your life and body shape.

EXPOSURE

- Expose yourself to play. Think about activities and places that you could put yourself in that you would be able to play in. Write a list of activities and places that you could try out.

BE ACTIVE

- Activity and movement is the easiest way to play and have fun.

GYM/MOVEMENT

- Play with your exercises, change them about, do them on one leg, on a bosu or swiss ball for example.
- Use the 'toys' in the gym – medicine balls, wobble boards, stability balls, kettlebells, cables, ropes etc.
- Warm-up with playful exercises and cool down with playful exercises
- If you are not enjoying your particular form of exercise, CHANGE IT!
- Functional training. This is the new type of training in gyms that uses toys mentioned above. It produces exercises that are functional, or relevant to everyday activities and that are in line with how you body was designed to move through evolution.

OTHER

- Sports - but don't take them too seriously!
- Play with pets - they bring out our playful side.
- Children – get down on the floor and let them lead you.
- Nourish your mode of play, and be with people who nourish it too.

"THE SUPREME ACCOMPLISHMENT IS TO BLUR THE LINE BETWEEN WORK AND PLAY."

ARNOLD TOYNBEE

UCS #4: WEIGHT GAIN IS HORMONAL

AT A GLANCE

This is the idea that excess weight, or more accurately, excess percentage body fat, is not simply a result of how much you eat and how little you exercise.

The body is evolutionarily predisposed to store body fat according to hormonal signals. Hormonal signals are controlled by the overall health of your body. The overall health of our body is controlled by a great deal more than how much you eat and how little you exercise!

YOU HAVE TO GET HEALTHY TO LOSE WEIGHT, NOT LOSE WEIGHT TO GET HEALTHY!

PALEO LENS

This is a hugely controversial topic, with many 'experts' and media outlets trying to persuade us that they have the answer but, one that is near impossible to scientifically validate due the un-measurable amount of variables. However, once again the paleo lens cuts through all of this to bring some clarity and simplicity.

Weight loss is not the simple equation of calories in and calories out. Body-fat percentage is regulated by our hormones in order to achieve the optimal performance necessary to survival in our current environment.

'Calories in, calories out' is simplistic nonsense and an insult to the sophistication of our bodies. We would not have survived millions of years of evolution if our bodies did not adapt to certain situations, storing fat when necessary, losing fat stores when appropriate.

Most obese people are actually malnourished. Their body is not receiving the right nutrients for optimum health and so sends hunger signals to the brain to keep eating. Similarly, many people are overweight because their body is under too much stress, stimulating too much adrenalin which suppress bodies 'rest & repair' functions such as digestion, sleep, blood sugar regulation. Exercise will release more adrenalin.

Have you ever wondered why some people never put on weight and some people can never lose it? This book is about understanding how our bodies really work; balancing our stressors for overall health, which in turn balances our hormones, thus leading to optimal weight and body fat stores throughout life. And note that this is all achieved without a painful, unnatural diet in sight!

WHAT ENVIRONMENT ARE YOU EXPOSING YOUR HORMONES TO?

Lack of calories = starvation = stress response
Poor nutrient content food = stress response

In both the scenarios detailed above, the body perceives a potentially life threatening situation, which thus triggers the stress response. We have to get healthy to balance our hormonal response.

SOME DETAIL

LOOKING THROUGH THE WRONG END OF THE TELESCOPE?

The simple equation to Weight loss – The Law of Thermodynamics

- Energy in versus energy out

The simplistic approach detailed above is espoused by diet companies, medical organisations, and governments the world over. It has one basic flaw…it simply does not work. The world is getting fatter with this advice.

SOME FIGURES FORM THE UK:

- 1,010,00 -The number of morbidly obese people in England
- 10% of six year olds are clinically obese. The number has tripled over the past 20 years.
- 4,619 obesity operations – gastric bands, balloons and stomach stapling – were carried out last year.
- £4.2bn Primary care trusts' obesity costs in 2007. Set to double by 2050.
- 1 billion - the number of overweight adults in the world. Some 300 million are obese.
- One in four Adults is obese; and nine in 10 will be overweight or obese by 2050.
- 9lbs – The average extra weight that a child carries now, compared with a child 20 years ago.
- 5,056 - The number of people admitted to hospital as a direct result of obesity in 2007-08.
- £600m – the size of the NHS drug bill for diabetes, the largest in primary care. Rising obesity has caused a sharp rise in type 2 diabetes.

(Statistics extracted from The Observer, "Who's to blame for Britain's obesity Epidemic?" 25.10.09)

In actual fact being overweight is our body's way of telling us that it is out of balance and that we need to change something in our lifestyle.

The statistics provide the evidence to show that a one-size-fits-all approach does not work for us humans. We are unique and need to listen to our bodies, and not the advertising, to create our own tailored healthy lifestyle.

THE SCIENCE BEHIND HEALTH

From a biological perspective, health is achieved by the body's ability to regenerate at a cellular level. The body turns over millions of cells every day, providing the energy for all the body's regulatory systems: nervous, hormonal, immune, thermal, reproductive, circulatory, digestive and eliminative.

If regeneration is compromised in any way, these systems will suffer, reducing an individual's ability to perform. Furthermore, the body is a cybernetic organism, a system of systems, meaning that if one system is compromised, all systems will be compromised.

Optimal cellular regeneration needs a positive balance of energy. This is achieved by ensuring a balance between the stressors in life to enable an individual to perform better.

See the 12 Week Programme Appendix IV for your own 'Energy Balance Audit'.

PRACTICAL IMPLEMENTATION

FOCUS ON HEALTH NOT WEIGHT LOSS

- Increase energy building behaviours
- Reduce energy depleting behaviours i.e. reduce stress load on the body
- See energy balance chart in 12-week programme (Appendix III)

EAT FOOD NOT FOOD PRODUCTS - Calories are an inappropriate focus when we are looking at nourishing the body. Look instead for

- Nutritionally dense food - for example, a fast food burger would not be considered nutritionally dense but a homemade burger might be.
- In supermarkets (or other food) compare price per nutrient rather than look of bulk (no formula for this just guesswork and intuition!).
- High quality – ideally local and organic
- A mix of vibrant colours in fruit and vegetables
- Short shelf life – reduced preservatives and higher nutrient value
- Foods in their most natural form – unprocessed, picked from the tress, pulled from the ground, fresh from the farm etc.

REAL FOOD DOES NOT USUALLY REQUIRE:

- An ingredients list
- Packaging
- Marketing

UCS #5:
EAT MORE FOOD & MORE FAT

AT A GLANCE

Rather than starving ourselves with calorie restriction diets, which is stressful to the body, we should plan to eat more food. This works on a number of levels:

- The food we choose will nourish our bodies, giving us all the nutrients we require for optimal health
- If our bodies are properly nourished we will eat less sugary, instant energy food. Real food allows us to sustain energy over a longer period of time

We should also eat more fat. Fat has been demonised on very shaky evidence, but is actually one of the keys to health and weight loss.

IF WE ARE OVERWEIGHT, WE ARE ACTUALLY STARVING - STARVING FOR THE RIGHT BALANCE OF NUTRIENTS THAT WILL INCREASE OUR METABOLIC RATE AND CONVERT THE FOOD WE ARE EATING INTO ENERGY INSTEAD OF STORING IT AS FAT.

PALEO LENS

The human body has been designed for times of food scarcity. Through evolution, in times of famine the body had to defend its weight fiercely. If we reduce the amount of food we consume, our bodies perceive this as a famine and slow down our metabolic rate accordingly. Even minimal weight loss of a pound a week will trigger this response.

"IN OTHER WORDS, THE LESS YOU EAT, THE LESS YOU NEED TO EAT BEFORE YOU START PUTTING ON WEIGHT AGAIN."

ROBERT WINSTON

What do you think made up a key component of our diet 10,000 years ago (and for millions of years before that)?

Answer 1: Kelloggs Special K, or
Answer 2: Organic saturated animal fat?

Eating fat does not make us fat. Fat is stored in your body, due to a hormonal response when insulin is released. Insulin is only released when blood sugar levels are elevated, which happens when carbohydrates high in sugar are eaten. It is carbohydrates, not fat, that cause body fat gains.

It takes 10,000 years for a human genome to evolve by 0.01%; so our bodies are near identical to when we were hunter-gatherers. During this period, our diets have changed beyond all recognition, with the advent of mass grain consumption, food processing and ever-increasing sugar consumption.

SOME DETAIL

Calorie restriction diets do not work because they change the profile in the cells to store more and burn less fat.

95% of people put back on the weight lost in a diet within 3 years
90% of these people put on more

'THE ONLY SCIENTIFICALLY GUARANTEED WAY TO PUT ON WEIGHT, IS TO GO ON A DIET'

Negative effects of calorie restriction diets include:

- Fat and protein deficiency
- Vitamin, mineral and enzyme deficiency
- Stress response
- Disrupted digestion (constipation/diarrhoea)
- Blood sugar imbalances
- Muscle wasting
- Mood swings
- Elevated insulin levels
- Muscles develop insensitivity to Insulin
- Fatigue which makes us reach for stimulants, which lead to further blood sugar and energy swings (coffee, chocolate, sweets)
- Increase lipogenic enzymes (fat storing) by 50%
- Decrease lipolytic enzymes (fat burning) by 50%
- Leads to weight gain, thus further dieting, and the vicious cycle repeats
- On each cycle we get progressively fatter!

NUTRIENT QUALITY

Calories are fairly irrelevant to a diet plan on a weight loss programme. Our focus should be on giving our bodies the right nutrients to function at optimal performance levels.

Do you think if we give our bodies all the right nutrients that we will crave further low nutrient, high sugar food?

THINK - DOES THIS FOOD NOURISH ME?

"ASIDE FROM THE VOLUMES OF LITERATURE STATING THE SUPERIORITY OF ORGANIC FOOD, POSSIBLY THE MOST COMPELLING EVIDENCE IS THAT OF YOUR OWN BODY. TRY EATING ORGANIC FOOD FOR A MONTH, OR EVEN BETTER, A YEAR AND DECIDE IF ORGANIC FOOD IS THE BETTER CHOICE FOR YOU AND YOUR FAMILY"

PAUL CHEK

METABOLIC EXPENSE

If you eat food with very low nutrient value it can actually mean the body has to use more energy to digest and eliminate these foods than the energy that the food gives the body. For example, in an experiment cows fed on a diet of straw died quicker than those fed nothing at all. We call these foods, displacement foods and are generally highly processed and or toxic food products.

EAT FOOD NOT FOOD PRODUCTS

FAT – DO NOT BELIEVE ALL THAT YOU HAVE BEEN TOLD

- Think of your *'paleo lens'* – we have been eating fat for 4 million years. This should give you at least a hint that it is not to blame for all society's ills!
- Do not expect 'fat' to be promoted - there is little profit in good quality fat, it is too expensive to produce and very difficult to add value to, because it is so good already.
- Eating fat does not cause heart disease. During the period of rapid increase in heart disease (1920-1960), American consumption of animal fats declined but consumption of hydrogenated and industrially processed vegetable fats increased dramatically. Animal fats contain many nutrients that protect against cancer and heart disease; elevated rates of cancer and heart disease are associated with consumption of large amounts of vegetable oil.
- As documented by recent publicity, a powerful sugar lobby in the 1970's was able to distort obesity research findings and blame fat instead of sugar for the problem.

THE BENEFITS OF EATING FAT

Fats are vital for their structural, functional and disease prevention properties.

They are:

- Concentrated and slow releasing sources of energy.
- Building blocks, especially for cell membranes and hormones.
- Hormone-like regulating substances (prostaglandins).
- Involved in the absorption of fat-soluble vitamins (A,D,E and K).
- Responsible for healthy nerve conduction.
- Involved in enhancing the immune system.
- Deficiencies in fats can lead to disease.

Sources of fats include oils, nuts, meat and cheese. Like the other macronutrients, fats are best in their natural form - how nature intended, rather than processed and packaged. It is because of the altering of the chemical properties of fats (processing) that they are now so maligned and misunderstood. This is compounded when eaten to excess.

BAD FATS

Of all substances ingested by the body, it is polyunsaturated oils that are most easily rendered dangerous by food processing, especially the unstable omega-3s. Examples of these oils include corn and vegetable oils.

Hydrogenation alters liquid unsaturated oil into a more saturated and solid at room temperature fat ('cis' to 'trans') with a longer shelf life. Examples of foods with hydrogenated fat include margarines, salad dressings, baked goods, ice cream, chocolate and many snack foods. Hydrogenated fat is potentially carcinogenic, disrupts normal metabolism, interferes with prostaglandin synthesis and is banned in many countries! Interestingly it was first introduced in 1912 and there was virtually no coronary heart disease before 1920! In fact heart disease was so rare that when a young internist named Paul Dudley White introduced the German electrograph (ECG) to his colleagues at Harvard University, they advised him to concentrate on a more profitable branch of medicine!

The new soft margarines or tub spreads, while lower in hydrogenated fats, are still produced from 'rancid' vegetable oils and contain many additives. So avoid them and eat butter.

THE RESEARCH

Many of the early studies into fats that led to the belief that fat, especially saturated fat, was unhealthy, did not distinguish between chemically altered fats and fats in their natural form. Furthermore, many of the studies can now be brought into question. An example of this is the 1948 Framington Heart Study, which is generally THE study always cited to prove that fat causes heart disease. The Director of this study admitted 40 years after its start that:

"THE PEOPLE WHO ATE THE MOST CHOLESTEROL, ATE THE MOST SATURATED FAT, ATE THE MOST CALORIES, WEIGHED THE LEAST." THE STUDY DID SHOW THAT THOSE WHO WEIGHED MORE AND HAD ABNORMALLY HIGH BLOOD CHOLESTEROL LEVELS WERE SLIGHTLY MORE AT RISK OF HEART DISEASE, BUT WEIGHT GAIN AND CHOLESTEROL LEVELS HAD AN INVERSE CORRELATION WITH FAT AND CHOLESTEROL INTAKE IN THE DIET. STOP! NOW READ THIS AGAIN – IT IS INCREDIBLY IMPORTANT.

Other studies have found that very low fat diets have led to an increase in deaths from cancer, brain haemorrhage, suicide and violent death.

Numerous epidemiological examples can be found that challenge the low fat recommendation. For example, The French Paradox, is a term used to 'explain' the relatively low levels of coronary heart disease in France, a country that has a diet that is loaded with saturated fats.

OMEGA 3

Omega 6 and omega 3 are called 'essential' fatty acids because they must come from our diet rather than being made in our bodies. Our ancestors ate these fats in a ratio of 50:50. Modern diets now consist of 3% Omega 3 and 97% Omega 6. Modern agricultural and industrial processes have reduced the amount of Omega 3 in commercially available vegetables, eggs, fish and meat. For example, organic eggs from hens allowed to feed on insects and green plants may contain a ratio of 50:50, but commercial supermarket eggs can contain as much as nineteen times more omega 6 than omega 3. However, take care with omega 3 oils as they are highly reactive and go rancid easily when exposed to heat and light. They should never be heated or used in cooking. Good omega 3 sources are fish, raw nuts & seeds.

A QUICK WORD ON CHOLESTEROL

Mother's milk is 55% cholesterol and it is made in the body, so it is hardly a dangerous substance! Cholesterol is a natural healing substance that steps in to repair damage in the blood vessels. Cholesterol is often seen as the bad guy, but this can be equated to blaming the fire brigade for the fire. Like saturated fats, the cholesterol we make and consume plays vital structural and functional roles in the body. However, damaged cholesterol (chemically altered) can damage arterial cells and build up plaque in arterial walls.

THERE IS NO LINK (AND NEVER HAS BEEN) BETWEEN CHOLESTEROL THAT YOU EAT AND CHOLESTEROL IN YOUR ARTERIES

COCONUT OIL

Coconut oil is fantastic source of saturated fat (92%). It has a large concentration of lauric acid, a medium-chain fatty acid that is especially effective against viruses and bacteria and strengthens the immune system. Interestingly lauric acid is also found in large quantities in mother's milk.

According to Bruce Fife, N.D., author of The Healing Miracles of Coconut, fatty acids found in coconut have proven to be effective in destroying the viruses that cause influenza, herpes, hepatitis C, and AIDS; the bacteria that cause pneumonia, food poisoning, urinary tract infections, and meningitis; fungi and yeast related to ringworm and candida; and parasites that cause intestinal infections.

THE BIG FAT CONCLUSION

- The scientific evidence when honestly evaluated does not support the conclusion that saturated fats cause heart disease.
- Saturated fats are good fats.
- Eating fat does not make you fat.
- Avoid processed fats especially margarines, polyunsaturated oils and other low-fat products.
- Eat high quality, unprocessed fats such as those found in meats, olive and coconut oils, nuts (preferably cracking the shell yourself), butter, cream, avocados and eggs.

PRACTICAL IMPLEMENTATION

Plan your meals in advance

Make extra food for leftovers

Have established channels for quality produce
- Organic box deliveries
- Known farm shops, butchers etc
- Local farms often deliver straight to your door
- Trusted shops
- Online companies

Find ways to get fat into difficult meals such as breakfast and snacks eg:
- Lots of butter (do not eat margarine)
- Coconut oil in smoothies
- Cream in coffee
- Heavy cream desserts to offset the chocolate/sugar
- Choose fattier cuts of meat as long as the quality is high – (see Toxic Fat section)
- Pate & crudités
- Never eat carbohydrates on their own, always mix with protein & fat
- Eat nutrient dense foods such as offal

If it wasn't here 10,000 years ago do not eat it
- Do not eat grains (bread, pasta, cereals etc)
- Limit your intake of sugar (remember 'ose' = sugar. Examples include lactose in milk, dextrose, fructose)

Go for low glycemic index carbohydrates e.g. above ground vegetables

Balance energy/blood sugar levels by eating regularly
- Start with 4-5 meals a day
- Use a food diary to monitor food eaten and timings

UCS #6:
ONE MAN'S FOOD IS ANOTHER MAN'S POISON

AT A GLANCE

Guess what? We are not all the same!

What is healthy for one person is not healthy for another. We have all read about populations that are really healthy because they all eat seaweed, or been told about a particular diet that worked for a friend. Well it may be great for them, but it may not be for you or me.

BIOCHEMICAL INDIVIDUALITY

Everyone has a different biochemical make-up; we are all unique and require a different balance of nutrients for optimal health.

WE CAN FIND OUT WHAT IS HEALTHY FOR US BY LISTENING TO OUR BODIES

PALEO LENS

Our dietary needs are largely determined by ancestral heritage. Our ancestors' dietary needs were a result of evolution and adaptation to the unique aspects of their natural habitat, including geographical location, climate, naturally occurring vegetation and available food sources.

As you can imagine, a diet that could effectively support the health of people living in one part of the world, say equatorial Africa, would be very different from a diet that could support the health of people in Nordic countries.

SOME DETAIL

BIOCHEMICAL INDIVIDUALITY

Dr Roger Williams, a world-renowned biochemist, identified over 60 years ago that biochemical individuality, the differences in anatomy and metabolism from person to person, has a significant impact on our health. For optimal function we each have unique nutritional needs and specific environmental requirements.

"THERE IS NO SUCH THING AS AN AVERAGE PERSON, WE ARE ALL GENETICALLY AND BIOCHEMICALLY UNIQUE. BUT WHEN THE SPERM MEETS, OUR CHARACTERISTICS ARE NOT LOCKED IN STONE. BAD GENES DO NOT CAUSE DISEASE BY THEMSELVES - NUTRITION AND ENVIRONMENT CAN ALTER THE OUTCOME."

Biochemical Individuality explains why:
- Some of us are better at detoxifying drugs and chemicals
- The harmful amino acid homocysteine, may or may not cause heart disease
- Cancer genes respond in different ways to diet and environment
- Some people are alcoholics or diabetics
- One person needs higher levels of a nutrient than another to be healthy

"(IT IS) MORE IMPORTANT TO KNOW WHAT SORT OF PATIENT HAS A DISEASE, THAN TO KNOW WHAT SORT OF DISEASE A PATIENT HAS"

SIR WILLIAM OSLER

WESTON A PRICE

In the 1930's, Dr Weston A Price, a dentist, studied isolated and primitive cultures and found that they were completely free of all the major degenerative diseases of modern civilizations. He also noted the different cultures ate different food and different macro-nutrient (carbohydrate, fat, protein) ratios. For example, the ratio of fats in the diet ranged from 30% to 80% with a large proportion of the Inuit diet coming from whale blubber.

A DIET THAT PROMOTES HEALTH AND VIGOUR IN ONE CULTURE CAN CAUSE SERIOUS ILLNESS IN ANOTHER.

"ONE MAN'S FOOD IS ANOTHER MAN'S POISON"

LUCRETIUS – QUOTED TWO THOUSAND YEARS AGO!

When Dr Price went back to these primitive cultures he noted that when they abandoned their native diets and adopted a western diet - with higher levels of grains and sugars - they developed the same chronic diseases now epidemic in modern societies!

He concluded that hereditary aspects play a major role in our dietary requirements; we are genetically programmed to require the same kind of foods as our ancestors depended upon for survival. However, with the cultural melting pots typical of modern society, it is hard to establish our hereditary dietary requirements.

Further complicating this situation, other factors also play a role in optimal diet, to include environmental conditions, specific nutrient deficiencies, and our level of stress or physical activity.

METABOLIC TYPING™

KEY PREMISE: ANY FOOD OR NUTRIENT CAN HAVE A VIRTUALLY OPPOSITE BIOCHEMICAL INFLUENCE ON DIFFERENT PEOPLE.

"THERE IS NO SUCH THING AS A HEALTHY DIET AND HAS NEVER HAD BEEN. THERE IS NOTHING INTRINSICALLY HEALTHY OR UNHEALTHY ABOUT ANY GIVEN FOOD. ALL THAT MATTERS IS HOW WELL A PARTICULAR FOOD OR DIETARY REGIMEN CAN FULFIL YOUR UNIQUE, GENETICALLY INHERITED METABOLIC REQUIREMENTS."

WILLIAM WOLCOTT

Metabolic Typing™ is a programme to help you customise your diet to your own unique body chemistry.

PRACTICAL IMPLEMENTATION

Realise that you are unique and have different nutritional requirements than others.

Be sceptical of any 'health' information about food product.

BE AWARE OF THE INTENTIONS AND EFFECTS OF FOOD COMPANIES' AND SUPERMARKETS' SALES AND MARKETING: REMEMBER THAT A GOOD SALES MODEL IS A ONE SIZE FITS ALL PRODUCT.

Once you remove poor quality food (generally high sugar, instant energy food) from your diet, you will be better placed to listen to your body to whether the food was right for you.

Use a food diary to monitor your reactions 1-2 hours after eating
- Are you still hungry, too full, jittery, have poor concentration, crave sweets, or are you satisfied with even energy levels?
- Experiment with different foods and vary the proportion of carbohydrates, fats and proteins

Be aware of your faeces – 'truly personal feedback!'
- Size, colour, smell, regularity

Ideally take a Metabolic Typing™ test and a food allergy test (Visit www.takeshapehealth.co.uk)

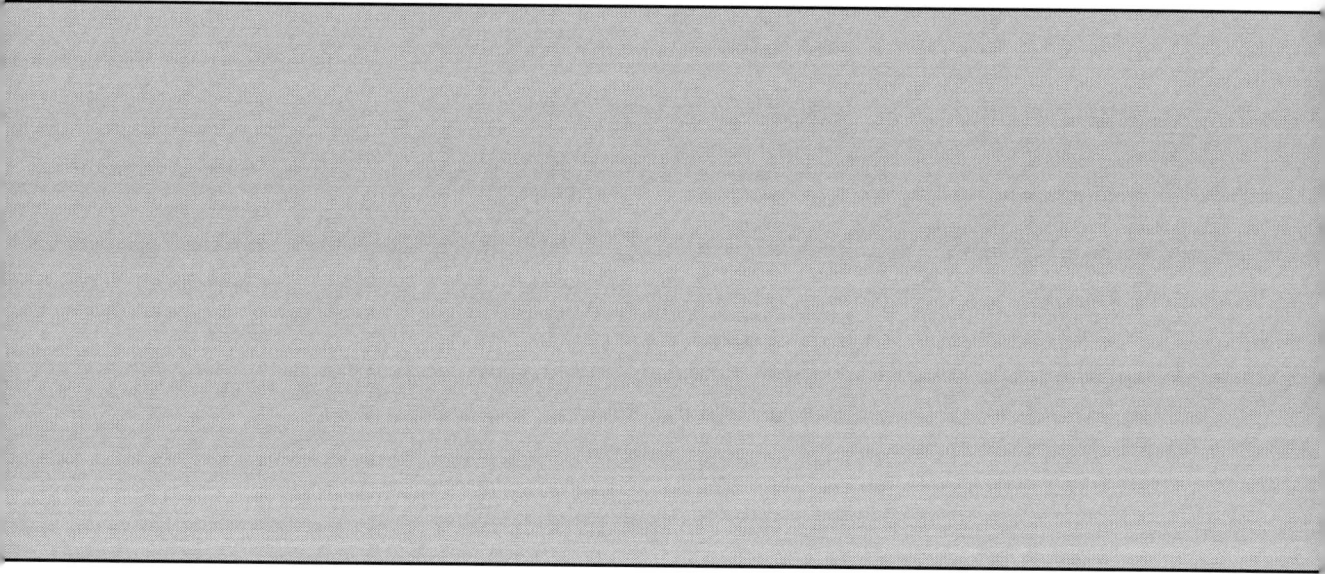

UCS #7:
WORK HARD, PLAY HARD, REST HARDER

AT A GLANCE

Sleep is biggest and best immunological defence scheme we have come up with. It also controls appetite and is therefore linked with factors such as obesity, type 2 diabetes and hypertension.

If we do not get over eight hours sleep a night, our bodies will crave carbohydrates to store as fat.

Furthermore, people are being stimulated for longer during the day, whether at work or play. This keeps our adrenalin levels too high for too long, creating a repair deficiency. Ours bodies can keep this up in the short to medium term, but this lack of rest and repair will eventually catch up with us leading to adrenal fatigue, illness and disease. Stress, whatever type, depletes from the same 'functional reserve' in the body. The answer is a reduction of all stressors and more rest.

Lack of sleep causes (NHS website 2014):
- Disruption of immune system
- Depression
- Anxiety
- Weight gain
- Type 2 diabetes
- Lower sex drive
- Heart disease
- Cancer (Wiley 2000)

PALEO LENS

WHY EXERCISING MORE AND EATING LESS CAN MAKE US FATTER

WHAT'S OUR BODY THINKING WHEN WE DO THIS? HOW ABOUT: "OH MY GOD A FAMINE'S COMING AND THERE'S A TIGER CHASING ME"

FAMINE - "SURVIVAL OF THE FATTEST"

Long days and short nights indicate to the body to eat lots of carbohydrates to store as fat for winter. It is the job of insulin to store excess carbohydrates as fat and cholesterol for hibernation.

TIGERS CHASING – "EXERCISE CAN MAKE YOU FAT!"

Running, jumping, climbing is akin to being chased which causes a stress response in the body. Cortisol is released and blood sugars are mobilised. Elevated blood sugars signal a release of insulin and over time lead to insulin resistance that causes fat storage and hypertension! This is how poorly structured exercise routines can make us fat.

SOME DETAIL

The balance between work and rest is very important and one many get wrong by working too hard with not enough rest.

NO-ONE ON THEIR DEATH-BED SAYS THEY WISH THEY WORKED MORE

STRESS AND THE AUTONOMIC NERVOUS SYSTEM (ANS)

SYMPATHETIC NERVOUS SYSTEM (SNS) "FIGHT/FLIGHT" RESPONSE:

- Shuts down viscera (organs) – which means there is no cellular growth, no turnover of cells, basically the bodies health functions being put on hold.
- Shuts down immune system which leads to an increase in opportunistic infections.
- Shuts off rational thinking – instead we use the instinctive brain which explains conditions like 'exam block'.
- Sends all energy to muscles.

"FOR OCCASIONAL USE ONLY"

ROBERT SAPOLSKY

PARASYMPATHETIC NERVOUS SYSTEM (PNS) "REST & REPAIR"

In this state the following functions are emphasised:
- Immune system
- Repair and growth
- Blood sugar regulation which in turn is key for bodyfat regulation
- Rational and creative brain
- Sex hormones production
- Sleep hormones production

- Circulation
- Digestion and Elimination
- Thermoregulatory systems

The SNS, should be for occasional use only. A sympathetically dominated person is likely to have some or all of the following symptoms: being overweight, lethargy, depression, anger, skin problems, frequents colds, difficulty relaxing, and insomnia. Interestingly, these symptoms are not generally recognised by the people who have them because they can take time to develop and because the sympathetic dominance provides the adrenalin to ignore these warning signs and get on with life.

CIRCADIAN RHYTHM

The most important part of our work / rest ratio is our circadian rhythm, our sleep wake cycle.

THE STATISTICS

Around 1910 the average adult would sleep between nine and ten hours a night. Now the average adult is lucky to get a full seven hours a night. Those numbers add up to an extra five hundred waking hours a year.

In nature we would sleep 4,370 hours out of a possible 8,760, or half of our lives. Eighty years ago we were down to 3,395 hours. Now we are lucky to get a measly 2,555.

In addition to this we are working longer with less leisure/hobby time.

OPTIMAL CIRCADIAN RHYTHM

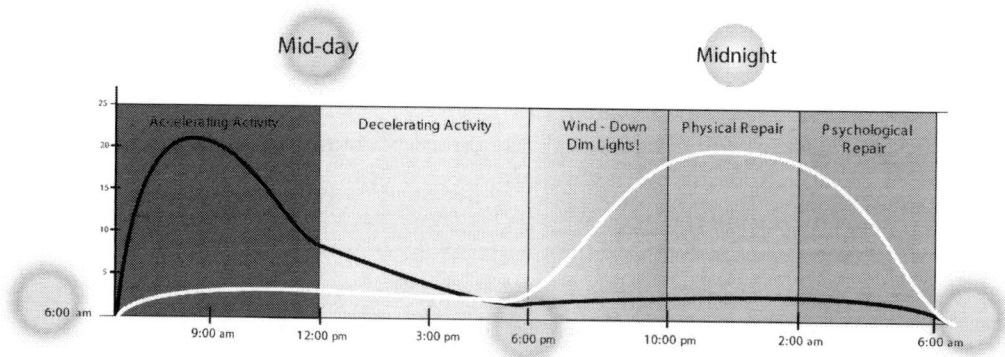

The black line above represents the adrenal stimulating hormone, cortisol.
The white line represents the sleep stimulating hormone, melatonin.

NORMAL 21ST CENTURY CIRCADIAN RHYTHM (SUB-OPTIMAL)

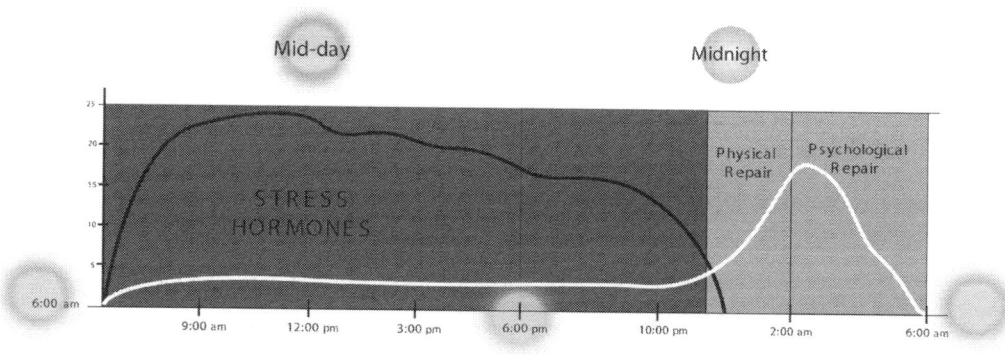

© Paul Chek, 1999. Diagrams reproduced with permission.

FAT STORAGE MODE

We should wake up hungry with low insulin and cortisol rising to deal with the stress of the day. If we have short nights of sleep this means insulin will stay higher during dark and cortisol falls so late it will not come up in the morning - a reversal of normal hormonal rhythms. With cortisol low and insulin still up, we are in fat storage mode.

In this state breakfast is easy to skip because with high insulin, we are not hungry. With low cortisol we may need an alarm to wake us up, and without the rise in cortisol we have no dopamine (see below), which means your day goes too fast and you're stupid! The only way to break this cycle is by getting to bed on time.

TIRED AND DEPRESSION

'A QUARTER OF AMERICANS ADMIT THEY ARE TIRED'

'121 MILLION PEOPLE IN WORLDWIDE ARE CHRONICALLY DEPRESSED (ONE IN 10 ADULTS)'

'ONE OUT OF EVERY 13 EUROPEANS IS CURRENTLY TAKING AN SSRI (SELECTIVE SEROTONIN REUPTAKE INHIBITOR) ANTIDEPRESSANT SUCH AS PROZAC TO COUNTER IT'

Serotonin and dopamine together control/balance primitive drives and emotions that govern sleep, mood, appetite, arousal, pain, aggression and even suicidal behaviour. If we do not get enough sleep they become out of out of balance.

Serotonin is the neurotransmitter in charge of impulse control. High serotonin means suppressed mood, withdrawal, defensiveness, Obsessive Compulsive Disorders, immobility (scared stiff, so no movement and therefore invisible to predators).

High serotonin levels are caused by excessive consumption of carbohydrates and the constant stimulus of lights. These two factors simulate the mating season for primitive humans. The mating season is a time of high stress and competition. This affects your mood negatively, making you feel sad because you live day and night as though you are under threat.

Dopamine on the other hand puts everything in sharp focus. Dopamine is so seductive because, with cortisol, it lays reward pathways for memory and time perception. This is why it is so hard to turn it off and go to bed. The blinking lights from video games, your computer, the TV are all addictive because of the dopamine release they cause.

'HIGH DOPAMINE LEVELS IS AN EXPERIENCE BETWEEN TAKING SPEED AND BEING IN LOVE'

WILEY

Our natural tendency to homeostasis means that we instinctively seek to balance things out. If we get too much of a good thing the receptor becomes resistant to the action of serotonin or dopamine and this is where the problems of low energy, tiredness and depression start.

Depression symptoms are responses to primal fear and panic resulting from high serotonin. Antidepressants work on serotonin levels through selective serotonin reuptake inhibitors (SSRI). They send serotonin levels over the top, block receptors and give us a more constant supply of serotonin. So the perceived danger is over, **as if** serotonin levels were really low.

BUT, THE WAY TO TURN 'AS IF' INTO REALITY IS TO TURN THE LIGHTS OUT.

PRACTICAL IMPLEMENTATION

Get over 8 hours sleep a night
- Reduce stimulation in the evening e.g. TV, computers, bright lights, phones
- Increase melatonin (sleep hormone) in the evening by cutting out / reducing stimulants / stimulating activities
- Have a bath, dim lights, use relaxation exercises, relaxation music, sleep promoting teas, meditation
- Get outside in day/sunlight during the day (especially between 12-3pm in winter) – this tells your bodies time clock when it is midday and so will know when it is midnight and therefore time to sleep.
- Balance blood sugars through diet (generally by reducing sugary carbohydrates and increasing fat - see UCS#5)
- Clear all sources of electromagnetic pollution as far away from your head as possible
- Control noise and light when asleep (e.g. black out curtains, rules for pets and children)
- Get up at the same time each morning (as close as possible to sunrise)
- Make changes slowly but consistently i.e. when bringing bedtime earlier do so ten-twenty minutes at a time

Use Energy building activities
- Tai Chi, yoga, CHEK zone exercises, meditation, gardening, laughing etc

High quality nutrition (see UCS#5)

Exercise in the morning or early afternoon only (ideally before 3-4pm) to avoid disrupting circadian rhythm (sleep/wake cycle)

Avoid caffeine after 3pm – limit yourself maximum of two maybe three cups of coffee/tea a day (the half-life of caffeine is six hours) to avoid disrupting circadian rhythm

Genuinely Rest
- Do not run on adrenalin the whole time
- Occasionally do nothing – notice that if, when you do nothing, you feel exhausted, you have some level of adrenal fatigue)
- Remember, you're a 'human being' not a 'human doer'
- This does not include watching TV!

UCS #8:
TOXIC FAT

AT A GLANCE

Any toxin our body ingests and then is unable to eliminate is stored, for safety this takes place as far away from our vital organs as possible. The furthest place is our fat stores.

The more toxic we are, the fatter we are.

Toxins are also major stressors to our body's regeneration systems, causing energy depletion and subsequent weight gain.

"CHEMICAL TOXINS ARE TO BLAME FOR THE GLOBAL OBESITY EPIDEMIC"

DR PAULA BAILLIE HAMILTON

PALEO LENS

Until a few hundred years ago, the human body was only exposed to organic compounds. Nowadays modern foods and water supplies expose the body to over 200 synthetic chemicals, and cosmetic products expose the body to a further 15-18,000 chemicals.

People in modern societies are continuously exposed to high concentrations of heavy metals. Metals like aluminium, cadmium, lead and mercury are commonly found in thousands of different food products, household products, personal products and untold numbers of industrial products and chemicals.

Heavy metals accumulate in the body's vital organs and tissues (e.g. brain, liver, kidneys, spleen, pancreas), thereby disrupting their ability to function normally. They also displace 'good' minerals (e.g. calcium, magnesium, zinc) that are necessary for vital enzyme reactions. In this way, heavy metals are often the primary cause of a very broad range of serious degenerative disorders and weight gain.

SOME DETAIL

Thousands of environmental toxins permeate every aspect of our air, food & water. They are unavoidable. These toxins invariably make their way into our bodies. For many of them, the body has no known detoxification mechanism. And even for things it can metabolise and get rid of, the quantities and combinations we are exposed to overwhelm our ability to detoxify the awesome amounts we accumulate each day. The result is that we slowly, silently, innocently stockpile these chemicals in our bodies.

"SINCE 1965 MORE THAN 4 MILLION DISTINCT CHEMICAL COMPOUNDS HAVE BEEN REPORTED IN THE SCIENTIFIC LITERATURE; OF THESE, 70,000 ARE IN COMMERCIAL PRODUCTION AND HAVE BEEN COMPLETELY UNTESTED OR INADEQUATELY TESTED, WHICH RAISES QUESTIONS ABOUT THEIR SAFETY"

DR SAMUEL EPSTEIN

THE FAT MAP OF GREAT BRITAIN

A report from Dr Foster Intelligence concluded that people living in northern industrial towns were fatter than those living in London or more rural areas of the UK. One factor causing this was exposure to hormone disrupting pollutants, often found in the industrial towns of the north where once there were mines, refineries, factories and tall chimneys, and where now there are chemical factories incinerators and waste transfer facilities regularly releasing toxins into the environment.

In developing nations there is a startling parallel between the rise of obesity and the rapid acceptance of urban/industrialised lifestyles.

2004 OBESITY: DEVELOPMENTAL ORIGINS AND ENVIRONMENTAL INFLUENCES

The US National Institute of Health made an urgent call for more research on the link between hormone disrupting chemicals and obesity, noting that exposure in adulthood and crucially, in the womb, can permanently disrupt the body's weight control mechanisms.

WEIGHT CONTROL

Our own natural weight control system is being poisoned by the toxic chemicals that we encounter in our every day lives. This damage makes it increasing difficult for our bodies to control weight, so we end up getting fatter, even if we eat less food.

Toxic synthetic chemicals are highly fat-soluble and when exposed to them the body creates fat to safely store those toxins it cannot process and eliminate safely. When dieting the body will not give up this fat easily as it would have to release the toxins back in the body, instead it prefers to lose muscle/lean weight.

Carbamates, a group of insecticides and herbicides used in the growing of food, cosmetic and medicinal ingredients are also used as growth promoter in battery-farm situations because they slow down metabolic rate. So the same synthetic chemicals used on our fruit and vegetables are used to fatten our livestock! Carbamates are also used in medicine to promote weight gain in humans.

Toxic chemicals, even when present in very small amounts, directly damage muscles and disrupt the hormones that control their growth. Toxins also affect the bodies own natural 'slimming' systems such catecholamine hormones.

THE TOXIC 21ST CENTURY – WHERE DO WE FIND THESE TOXINS?

- Chemicals in processed food, drinks, clothing & beauty products
- Pharmaceutical & recreational drugs
- Synthetic insecticides, pesticides, fungicides, fertilisers, hormones and antibiotics
- Radiation, car fumes, electromagnetic discharges
- Toxins in household goods
- Polluted air & water

"THE AMOUNT OF SYNTHETIC CHEMICALS MANUFACTURED IN THE UNITED STATES HAS INCREASED DRAMATICALLY OVER THE PAST HALF-CENTURY. IN THE U.S., OVER 75,000 INDUSTRIAL CHEMICALS ARE ON THE MARKET. UNFORTUNATELY, REGULATORS HAVE VERY LITTLE INFORMATION TO DETERMINE THE DANGER POSED BY THESE CHEMICALS. TENS OF THOUSANDS OF INDUSTRIAL CHEMICALS ON THE MARKET HAVE NOT BEEN TESTED FOR DEVELOPMENTAL HEALTH EFFECTS AT LOW DOSES. NO PUBLIC HEALTH INFORMATION EXISTS FOR CLOSE TO HALF OF THE HIGH PRODUCTION-VOLUME CHEMICALS. THE NEWLY-DISCOVERED CONNECTIONS BETWEEN CHEMICALS AND DISEASE OUTLINED HERE JUST BEGIN TO SCRATCH THE SURFACE OF THE POTENTIAL IMPACT OF CHEMICALS ON PUBLIC HEALTH."

GROWING UP TOXIC

"A WELL FUNCTIONING ADAPTATION CAPABILITY IS NEEDED TO OVERCOME CIVILISATION DANGERS. ALL INDUSTRIAL DANGERS ARE INCREASING. POLLUTION FROM CARS INVOLVES NANO PARTICLES, WHICH ARE HIGHLY DANGEROUS, AS THE BODY HAS NO FILTER TO PROTECT ITSELF FROM THESE. THIS IS MUCH MORE DANGEROUS TO HUMAN HEALTH THAN CIGARETTES. NANO PARTICLES, TO WHICH THE BODY IS NOT ADAPTED, ARE THE REAL CANCER CAUSING PARTICLES. LIVING IN LONDON IT IS EQUIVALENT TO SMOKING 200 CIGARETTES A DAY."

DR KUCERA

COSMETICS

UP TO 60 PERCENT OF WHAT WE BATHE IN OR PUT ON OUR SKIN IS INGESTED INTO OUR BODIES.

We readily accept that skin patches, such as nicotine patches, work by absorption through the skin and that some medications are applied under the tongue for rapid absorption however, we do not always think what is in our toothpaste, hair and skin care products.

Ingredients to avoid: Sodium laurel sulphate (SLS), Parabens, PEG's, Fluoride, Propylene, Glycol, Aluminium chlorohydrate to name but a few.

Be aware 'organic' in cosmetics does not mean the same as in food. Cosmetic products can be labelled organic when only 70% of its ingredients are organic, leaving a massive 30% of ingredients which could be harmful. Food, to be labelled organic, has to be 100% organic.

ELECTRO-MAGNETIC (ELM) POLLUTION

There are many different theories on how electromagnetic radiation interacts with our bodies, but pulsed microwave radiation, such as that used by wifi and mobile phones is thought to affect our body's cells in an unnatural way.

Our body's cells interpret the slow vibrations of these microwaves as a foreign invader and close down the cell membrane, impairing the flow of nutrients into the cell and waste products out of the cell. It also disrupts intercellular communication, a key feature in balancing our health.

Non-thermal effects of microwave radiation include changes to the blood brain barrier, an increase in the production of cancer causing free radicals, a decrease in body melatonin (the sleep hormone) and the disruptions in intra-cellular communication. The wifi industry's products have come to market without having to undergo any trials.

"IF YOU ARE A DRUG COMPANY MARKETING A NEW DRUG, YOU GO THROUGH YEARS OF TESTING TO PROVE YOUR PRODUCT IS SAFE, IF YOU ARE A WIFI DEVELOPER YOU DO NOT NEED TO PROVE ANYTHING"

PROFESSOR DENIS HENSHAW

The evidence is well documented but there appears little desire by the 'powers that be' to do anything that might slow down the rate of growth in this industry. The public exposure to electro-magnetic pollution has exceeded everyone's expectations and more technology is being marketed every day.

PRACTICAL IMPLEMENTATION

REDUCE CONTACT WITH TOXINS

- Organic & natural food (especially meat)
- Organic & natural health & beauty products
- Organic & natural cleaning products

BREATHE CLEAN AIR

- Get out into the country side
- Buy house plants to clean indoor air
- Open windows in cars & houses

DE-TOXIFY

- Hot/cold showers
- Saunas
- Detox. Teas
- Drink purified water (Amount = your body weight in kg's x 0.033)

GO BAREFOOT ON THE EARTH

Literally earthing the body, dumping electrical charge (See UCS#2)

LOSE WEIGHT

Do this slowly and incrementally - we can feel awful when we lose percentage bodyfat, because we are releasing toxins back into our bloodstream

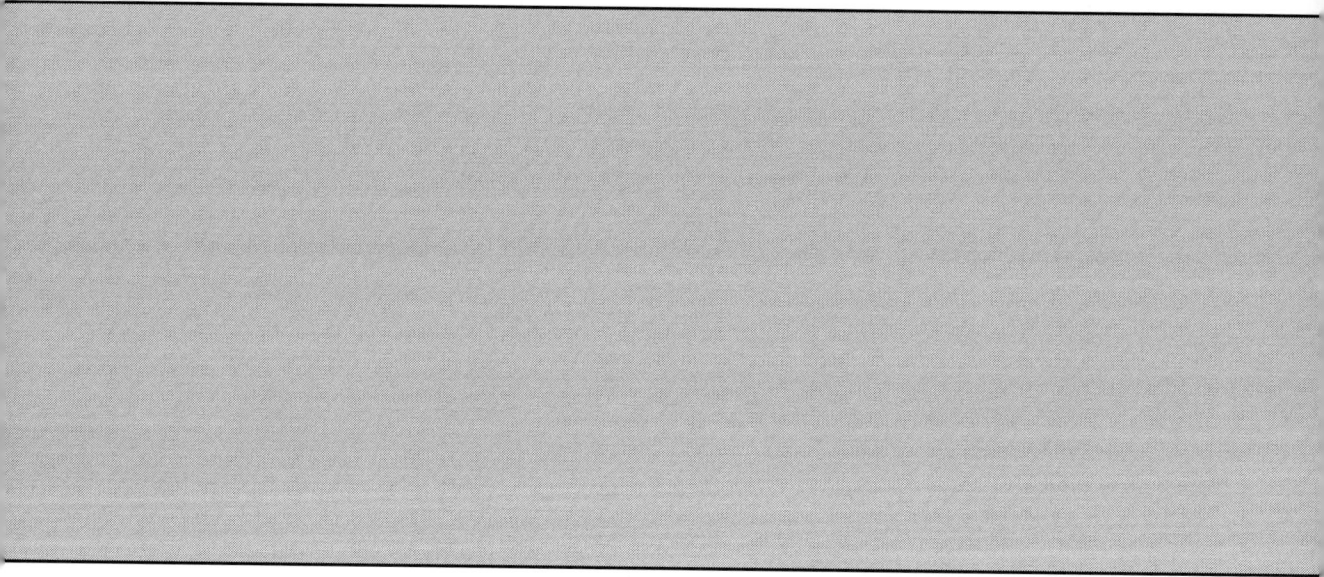

UCS #9
USE YOUR MIND, ALL OF IT

"MOST OF OUR PROBLEMS ARE RELATED TO THE MIND, SO WE HAVE TO WORK TO REDUCE ARE DESTRUCTIVE EMOTIONS"

DALAI LAMA

AT A GLANCE

We have already noted that the body is a highly complex system of systems (cybernetic or holistic). For example, weight loss is not as simple as calories in and calories out. It is the mind that influences the physical either consciously or unconsciously.

It is estimated that only 5% of the mind is conscious and 95% is unconscious. This is why New Year's resolutions rarely work. We consciously commit to the resolution but, as this is only 5% of mind, the other 95% carries on running your life as before.

The key to change is tapping into the unconscious mind. One of the easiest ways to do this is to have, and write down a dream. By doing this you emotionalise, which mobilises your unconscious towards your goals.

PALEO LENS

Cells come together into a community for a greater chance of survival but the pay off is that they have to conform. Cells defer their belief system to a central command, the brain.

NEGATIVITY – A PRIMAL WAY OF BEING

Throughout evolution, there were a lot of challenges to our survival such as predators. It made survival sense for our brain to be attuned to the negative and have an automatic response to danger.

AUTOMATIC BEHAVIOUR & CHUNKING KNOWLEDGE

We have four billion nerve impulses per second in the brain but we are only conscious of two thousand of them. This means most of our behaviour is automatic. Think of a time you have driven home deep in conversation with a good friend; your conscious was engaged in deep conversation and you have no idea how you got home. Now think of the complexity of driving when you first learnt including arm and leg co-ordinated movements, 360 degree vision, complex decisions about steering, pull-outs and predicting other road users! With learned experience you relegate these complex activities into your unconscious in what sports psychologists call chunking.

CHUNKING

Putting together learned knowledge in chunks which act as building blocks that new learned knowledge can be built upon.

SOME DETAIL

We are so conditioned to a daily routine, it appears we have no control or choice over what we do or experience. We repeat the same patterns i.e. resolutions, diets, health drives, relationships etc.

If you do not get to your core belief your, thoughts and actions are not on the same level. The world has everything but you can only see what you are trained to see. You find what you look for.

THE LAW OF ATTRACTION:

'YOU ARE A LIVING BEING AND YOU INEVITABLY ATTRACT INTO YOUR LIFE, THE PEOPLE, CIRCUMSTANCES, IDEAS AND RESOURCES IN HARMONY WITH YOUR DOMINANT THOUGHTS.'

Have you ever noticed:
- That your friends are like you
- Partners often look similar in appearance
- People repeat the same mistakes

This is because like attracts like.

YOU GET EXACTLY WHAT YOU ASK FOR...

If you think all the time about wanting to lose weight, that is exactly what you get, 'wanting to lose weight' (never actually losing it, just the 'wanting' to lose it).

Treat the unconscious like a five-year old child. It, like a child, does not understand negatives and nuances. If you say to a child "don't touch that" all they hear is "touch that". You must ask for exactly what you want in positive language.

POSITIVE VOLITION NOT THINK POSITIVE

Positive thinking is generally just a thin veneer disguising the negative. Positive volition is a positive decision on a course of action and goes deeper into the unconscious, obtaining better results.

For example, rather than a New Year's resolution to lose weight, list a number of positive actions that you can do (such as the 12 Week Programme at the end of this book).

BE PRESENT

Focus on the here and now. It is all we have, everything else, past and future is our mind creating. It is very easy to make ourselves unhappy. It is our tendency to 'add on' to an experience e.g. a bus is late and we get all worked up. However, by being aware of our thoughts and our unconscious, primal reactions, we can control our emotions for better outcomes.

CASE STUDY

I had a client who, as I got to know him in training, told me about his dealings with other people in the business that he ran. More often than not these were about falling out with a customer or supplier and obviously it was always the other person's fault! Alarm bells went off in my unconscious and sure enough our relationship ended in the same way as many other of his business dealings.

The client was doing really well losing lots of weight and getting really fit for a marathon. He was even telling everyone he came into contact how wonderful I was! However, his results were starting to plateau (as he was not able or willing to follow all the lifestyle advice), and it was coming up to the time to re-sign for some more personal training. Rather than make the decision himself, he unconsciously engineered a situation where it was some else's fault (mine!) that he was not able to continue his health and fitness drive.

There are a few points here:
- Behaviour repeats itself in all areas of life work, personal
- We choose what happens to us
- If we blame someone else for our situation, stop and think
- My client's results were plateauing because he was not ready to take on the ideas in this book, particularly the chapter on 'rest'

- It is interesting that however much I tried to rationalise the events, my emotional mind kept getting annoyed and questioning my behaviour. What helped me was my core values, in particular looking after my own energy and health before I can help others

DREAM / LEGACY

Goals are about getting somewhere, about achieving. But what happens if we do not achieve our goal? Even worse, what happens when we achieve our goal? Are we now happy? Have the goal posts moved? Do we need to set more goals? What happens when we achieve the new goal?

Instead of goals, which might or might not work, we need to think of something bigger, something really important, something that galvanises every cell into the direction that we want our life to go. A dream or a legacy does this. A legacy is what we are going to leave behind when we are gone. Although the word, legacy, conjures up thoughts of death it is, obviously, more about what we do when we are alive. It is how do we want to be remembered.

WHAT WOULD YOU LOVE TO CREATE?

Have you ever thought of this? Have you ever written it down? It is a very powerful motivator when we do. It gives clarity and purpose to every fibre in our body, mobilising our unconscious.

Interestingly, top sports people find it easier to fail at their chosen goal (generally in hindsight) than to achieve it. By failing, their life has a clear focus and purpose - to get better, to train harder and to win 'gold'. But by winning 'gold', their life's purpose has just been taken from them.

If we are able to create and live by our dreams they are real now, and ongoing. Goals are about achieving something because we think it will make us happy. A dream or legacy is about the energy of happiness that attracts good things into our life. The here and now is what are important, because the present is all we have, the past and the future are just creations and perceptions of the mind.

PRACTICAL IMPLEMENTATION

HAVE A DREAM / LEGACY AND WRITE IT DOWN

- This is a great way to tap into our sub conscious/ emotional mind rather than just the 5% conscious mind
- What would you love to create?

BE PRESENT

- Live in the now, not the past or the future
- 5% in the past, 15% in the future, 80% in the present

BE AWARE OF YOUR THOUGHTS

- If we are stressed acknowledge this
- Brings us into the present, the now

HAVE POSITIVE VOLITION

- Remember our unconscious does not understand negatives

BE AWARE OF WHAT WE SAY

- Positive / negative
- What we say about others is more a reflection on us rather than others
- And, in this way, do not take anything personally
- What you dislike in other people is what you tend to dislike most in yourself
- Gossip always comes round to bite you

GRATITUDE

- Practise thanks for what you have and for what you want as if you already have it

LEARN TO MEDITATE

- There are plenty of classes, courses, apps & audio to help you do this

DO OUR BEST

- Our best is always good enough
- It will constantly change
- And you will avoid self-judgement, self-abuse & regret

WORRY NOT

- If there is something you can do about it, do it. If not, 'don't worry'

OTHER HELP / TECHNIQUES

- Psyche-K, NLP, EFT, counselling

UCS #10
NURTURE WINS
OVER NATURE

AT A GLANCE

Many people, fuelled by the media think that health and weight is determined by their DNA – "it's all in the genes!" The media is always talking about certain genes that store fat, carry disease and the like.

However, I've got bad news for you, you cannot blame your genes. It is your environment and subsequent learned behaviour, which controls your body and your life.

This means that you can choose your actions and your thoughts, which determine your feelings and physiology.

YOU GET TO CHOOSE - INDIRECTLY YOU CHOOSE YOUR PHYSIOLOGY (YOUR BODY & FEELINGS) BY YOUR ACTIONS AND YOUR THOUGHTS.

PALEO LENS

"THRIVAL OF THE FITTINGINGEST"

LIPTON

Evolution occurs in the context of environment not separate from it. The process can be seen as an environment constantly seeking to rebalance itself. In biology 'fit' actually means how well an organism 'fits' its environment. Those that fit best, survive.

Darwinism states that genes only change at random, however, this is not entirely true. Lamarck's evolutionary theory states that we adapt to changes in the environment. This means that we are not a slave to our genes, we get to change according to our perceptions of our surroundings.

Published in the Nature journal in 1988 Cairns' 'directed mutations' research proved that environmental stimuli could feed back into an organism and direct a rewriting of genetic information.

Why do we not know about this? Because it is at odds with so much of what was already 'known' in science and what we believed to be the truth. Ironically, Cairns' research was labelled as 'heresy'.

"WHEN A GENE PRODUCT IS NEEDED, A SIGNAL FROM ITS ENVIRONMENT, NOT AN EMERGENT PROPERTY OF THE GENE ITSELF, ACTIVATES THE EXPANSION OF THAT GENE."

HF NIJHOUI

So, the behaviour we are expressing is a reflection of the outside and is not controlled by genes but by perception.

PERCEPTION = INTERNAL ENVIRONMENT, EXTERNAL ENVIRONMENT & BELIEF

SOME DETAIL

PRIMACY OF ENVIRONMENT & EPIGENICS

The new science of Epigenics, which literally means 'above genes', proves that our environment and subsequent behaviour control which genes 'switch on' in our body and which do not.

The flow of information in biology (at a cellular level) starts with an environmental signal, then goes to the regulatory protein and only then goes to DNA, RNA and the end result a protein. It is the protein that controls behaviour of the cell and therefore the behaviour of an organism i.e. you and me.

CHOICE THEORY

"WE CHOOSE EVERYTHING WE DO"

WILLIAM GLASSER

We choose all our **ACTIONS & THOUGHTS**
And indirectly our **FEELINGS & PHYSIOLOGY**

The only person's behaviour we can control is our own. All we can get from other people is information. How we deal with information is our choice.

RELATIONSHIPS

Generally all long-standing psychological problems are relationship problems. The relationship is always part of our present lives. What happened in the past that was painful has a great deal of what we are today but revisiting this painful past can contribute little or nothing to what we need to do now. Improve an important current relationship.

NEEDS

We are driven by five genetic needs: survival, love (and belonging), power, freedom and fun. These needs have to be satisfied - they can be delayed but not denied. Only we can decide when they are satisfied no one can tell us. We can't satisfy others needs. We can satisfy these needs only by satisfying a picture in our quality worlds - the most freedom we experience is when we satisfy a picture in our quality worlds. Our quality world is what we think is important and can be defined by our values.

BEHAVIOUR

All we can do from birth to death is behave - all behaviour is total i.e. acting, thinking, feeling and physiology. All behaviour is designated by verbs – e.g. I am choosing to depress and not I am depressed. All total behaviour is chosen but we only have active control over acting and thinking.

LOVE YOURSELF

In our world/culture to love ourself is often used with negative connotations for example we say that 'he loves himself' or 'she loves herself' about someone we perceive to be arrogant, beautiful, or aloof. However, self-love is the most important thing you can do for your health and happiness.

HOW CAN YOU EXPECT ANYONE TO LOVE YOU IF YOU DO NOT EVEN LOVE YOURSELF?

If you really loved your body would you not
- Only provide it with nourishing food?
- Make sure you could recover from any stressor, exercise or other?
- Focus on its good points and not its bad points (giving the good points energy)?
- Make sure it gets proper rest?

In coaching we use the '**I, We, All**' model. The 'I' is yourself, the 'We' is you and your partner, the 'All' is everyone else (children, family, friends, colleagues). The concept is that we must first look after ourselves before we can look after our partner, and we must look after ourselves and our partners before we can look after anyone else.

AIRPLANE ANALOGY

"IN AN EMERGENCY PUT ON YOUR OWN OXYGEN MASK FIRST BEFORE HELPING OTHERS"

This concept is often hard for a mother to take on board at first. Often, they look after their children's priorities before their own, but this does not work for a number of reasons:

Firstly, to be able to look after children properly we need energy, health and vitality. If the mother is not looking after her needs first and not eating well, resting well, exercising, and happy, she will not have the energy to look after her children.

Secondly, children learn most of their behaviour by observation and copying. If the mother is overweight, lacking energy and generally not looking after herself this will be the example the children will copy no matter how many times the mother might tell the children what to do. Meal times is a very simple example; it is much more powerful to 'eat your own greens' and not try and force greens down a child. Any parent who has tried to coerce a child into eating something they perceive to be healthy knows that it generally involves the opposite of the desired reaction. Generally, by observation of the parent, the child will come round to eating the healthier food. If they do not come round the food might not be right for the child's metabolic type and so should not be forced.

CORE VALUES

Our values determine how we choose to invest our time, our energy and our money. They also define our needs relative to our wants. Values need to be written down so that they can be reinforced and amended.

Values will include:
- What, where and when will we feed ourselves
- What are we willing to spend time studying
- Who are we willing to work for (whose dreams we will contribute to!)
- What religious beliefs you will invest your energy into
- How much of a consumer relative to a generator of resources we choose to be

Are you living to your values or your parents values?

The life you want to lead or the ones you think your parents want you to lead?

When we choose our own values, we become self-aware and free. For many, even and especially people in healthcare, there is a lack of congruency between what people teach and what they do. When our life is in line with our core values it makes us very aware of and resilient to what drains our vitality. It means we will become ill less and will recover more quickly when we do. It is also key to our happiness and wellbeing.

PRACTICAL IMPLEMENTATION

CHOOSE HAPPINESS

- Put happiness as a realistic life goal
- The turning towards happiness as a valid goal and the conscious decision to seek happiness in a systematic manner can profoundly change the rest of our lives.

CHOOSE TO LOVE YOUR BODY

- Tell yourself five times in the mirror each morning that you love yourself
- Or have a daily ritual such as in the shower going over your body and feeling love for every part

IMPROVE AN IMPORTANT CURRENT RELATIONSHIP

WRITE DOWN YOUR VALUES

- See how your life is in tune with your values
- If they are out of tune you will not be happy

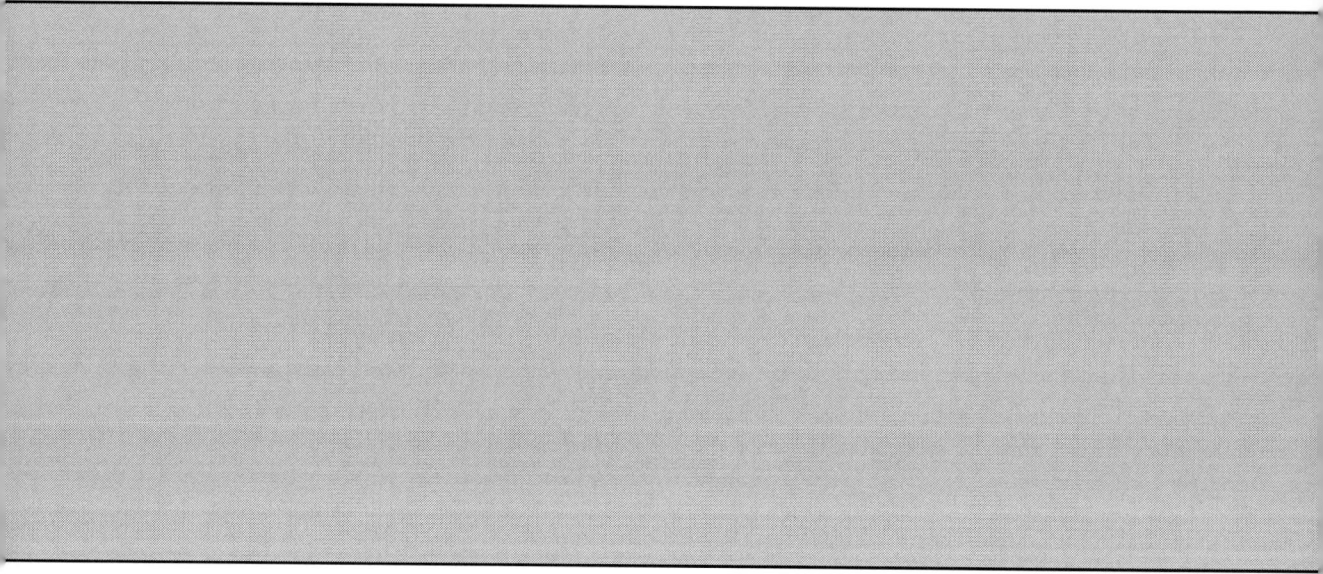

SUMMARY

IT'S PRETTY EASY REALLY...

1   Move your body every day

2   Go barefoot

3   Enjoy it

4   Get healthy to lose weight (not the other way round)

5   Eat fat (it doesn't make you fat)

6   Personalise your diet by listening to your body

7   Sleep well

8   Reduce toxic load on your body

9   Write down your dream life/body

10 Actively choose the body you want

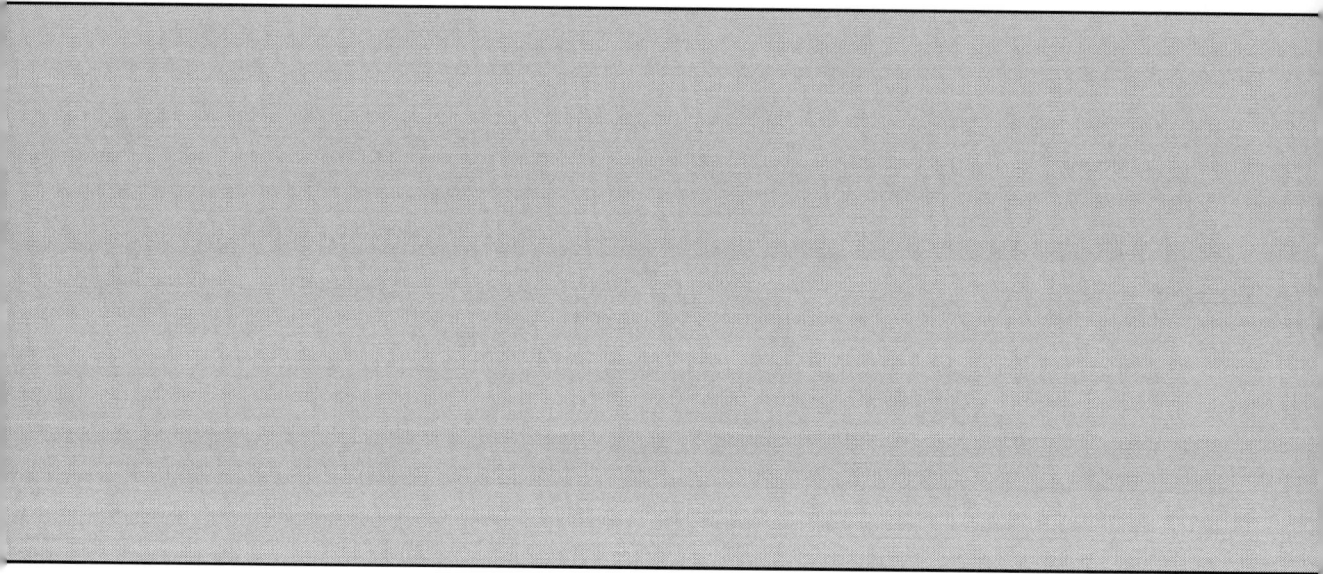

APPENDIX I
FOOD
INTOLERANCES

Eating food is putting a foreign substance into your body meaning your immune system will have some level of response/activity. If you have eaten the same food everyday of your life you will probably have an intolerance to it. The body likes variety!

Two key foods to avoid or at least test for intolerance are gluten and dairy.

The most simple intolerance test – remove the food totally from your diet for two weeks then after two weeks have the food and see how it makes you feel. If you have any adverse reactions you will have an intolerance to that food

GLUTEN

- wheat
- barley
- flour
- bread
- cereal
- pasta
- rye
- couscous
- cakes, biscuits
- stuffing
- sausages
- malt
- starch
- whisky
- beer
- malt vinegar
- bran
- bulgar
- semolina
- pizza
- noodles

Read the ingredients it's in many things you wouldn't expect!

I don't recommend buying 'gluten-free' products such as 'gluten-free' bread, biscuits, cake etc. because you are missing the point about only eating food that nourishes you and the alternative is often worse (different but often more intolerable).

DAIRY

Note the two parts of milk the buttermilk and the lactose. Buttermilk is the fat, used for butter and generally people can tolerate this. Lactose is the sugar ('ose' = sugar) and is the part of milk people generally have an intolerance to.

PASTEURISATION

De-natures the milk making it harder for the body to digest. Many people can tolerate unpasteurised or 'raw' dairy such as cheeses and creams.

- Milk
- Yoghurt
- Butter
- Cheese
- Ice cream
- Cream
- Ghee
- Whey (hydrolysed or other)
- Casein

Other foods to avoid:

SOYA

- Lecithin
- Miso
- Tempeh & tofu
- Soya beans
- Soya protein
- (look for in a high percentage of processed foods)

MSG (MONO SODIUM GLUTAMATE) E621/E622 "FLAVOUR ENHANCER"

- chicken nuggets
- fish fingers
- sausages
- pork pies
- Chinese take-away
- crisps
- soya sauce
- stock cubes
- tinned beans, sweetcorn, mushrooms
- flavour enhancers

SUGAR

- corn syrup
- fruit juices
- golden syrup
- maltose
- molasses and treacle
- dextrose (corn sugar)
- malt syrup
- sucrose
- lactose (milk sugar)
- fructose (fruit sugar)
- glucose (corn sugar)
- inert syrup
- maple syrup

APPENDIX II
HEALTH
QUESTIONNAIRE

UCS#1 HIT OR NEAT

Do you move your body for at least 30 mintes every day?
- ☐ Yes
- ☐ No (10 points)

What intensity do you 'mostly' train at?
- MHR = Maximum Heart Rate
- RPE = Rating of Perceived Exertion – 1 to 10 scale how hard does your exercise feel with 1 being very easy and 10 being very, very hard)
- ☐ 95% or 9/10 RPE
- ☐ 70-90% MHR or 6-9 RPE (10 points)
- ☐ 51-70% MHR or 6-7 RPE (5 points)
- ☐ 50% MHR or 5 RPE or less

Do you have back pain?
- ☐ Yes at moment (10 points)
- ☐ Yes in the last 5 years (5 points)
- ☐ No

UCS#2 LESS IS MORE, FOOTWISE

Do you wear conventional trainers when moving?
- ☐ Yes (10 points)
- ☐ Sometimes (5 points)
- ☐ No

Do you have a repetitive strain sporting injury?
- ☐ Yes (10 points)
- ☐ No

UCS#3 HAVE FUN

Is your exercise enjoyable?
- ☐ Yes, always
- ☐ Yes mostly (5 points)
- ☐ Yes, sometimes (10 points)
- ☐ No (20 points)

UCS#4 WEIGHT GAIN IS HORMONAL

Have you been on a calorie restriction diet before?
- ☐ Yes 5x or more (10 points)
- ☐ Yes 2-4 times (5 points)
- ☐ Yes once (1 point)
- ☐ No

Does you eat processed food?
- ☐ Yes (10 points)
- ☐ No
- ☐ Occasionally (5 points)

Do you worry or get anxious?
- ☐ Yes, all the time (10 points)
- ☐ Sometimes (5 points)
- ☐ No

Is your sex drive lower than normal for you?
- ☐ Yes (10 points)
- ☐ No

UCS#5 EAT MORE FOOD & MORE FAT

Do you eat carbohydrates on the own eg. sweets, cakes, biscuits?
- ☐ Yes (10 points)
- ☐ Rarely (5 points)
- ☐ No

Do you avoid fatty foods?
- ☐ Yes (10 points)
- ☐ No

Do you feel hyper-active and/or lethargic during the day?
- ☐ Yes (10 points)
- ☐ Sometimes (5 points)
- ☐ No

Do you buy meat, fruit and vegetables that are generally:
- ☐ Organic / grass-fed/ traditional / seasonal?
- ☐ Standard supermarket? (8 points)
- ☐ The cheapest? (10 points)

UCS#6 ONE MAN'S FOOD IS ANOTHER MAN'S POISON

Is your diet unique to you?
- ☐ Yes
- ☐ No (10 points)

Do you know how food makes you feel?
- ☐ Yes
- ☐ No (10 points)

Do you eat gluten & pasteurised dairy?
- ☐ Yes, both (10 points)
- ☐ Yes only one (5 points)
- ☐ No

UCS#7 WORK HARD, PLAY HARD, REST HARDER

How many hours sleep a day you generally get?
- ☐ 8 or more
- ☐ about 7 (5 points)
- ☐ less than 6 (8 points)
- ☐ less than 4 (10 points)

Do you meditate, yoga, tai chi or similar?
- ☐ Every day (minus 10 points)
- ☐ 5x / wk (minus 8 points)
- ☐ 1-4x / wk (minus 5 points)
- ☐ No

How much time do you spend outside each day in daylight?
- ☐ 5 or more hours (minus 10 points)
- ☐ 1-4 hours
- ☐ 1 hour (5 points)
- ☐ 20 minutes (8 points)
- ☐ none (10 points)

Do you get ill when you have a holiday?
- ☐ Yes, often (10 points)
- ☐ Yes, sometimes (5 points)
- ☐ No

Do you feel tired when you stop doing stuff?
- ☐ Yes (10 points)
- ☐ No

How many cups of coffee do have a day
- ☐ 3 or more (10 points)
- ☐ 1-2 before 3pm (3 points)
- ☐ none

UCS#8 TOXIC FAT

What is your measurement around your middle (tummy button level)?
- ☐ Over 100cm (10 points)
- ☐ 80-100cm (5 points)
- ☐ Under 80cm

Do you wake up around 3am in the middle of the night?
- ☐ Yes (10 points)
- ☐ Sometimes (5 points)
- ☐ No

Are you sensitive to pollutants?
- ☐ Yes (10 points)
- ☐ Sometimes (5 points)
- ☐ No

Hydration – do you drink?
- ☐ 2-4 litres per day of filtered water and non caffeinated teas
- ☐ Less than 2 litres (5 points)
- ☐ Generally only tea, coffee, carbonated or sugary drinks (10 points)

UCS#9 USE YOUR MIND – ALL OF IT

What percentage of your thoughts are negative
- ☐ 95% (10 points)
- ☐ 70% (8 points)
- ☐ 50% (5 points)
- ☐ 30% (3 points)
- ☐ 0%

Are you aware that your body and your life situation is of your choosing?
- ☐ Yes
- ☐ No (10 points)

Do you have your dream/legacy written down?
- ☐ Yes
- ☐ No (10 points)

UCS#10 NURTURE WINS OVER NATURE

Is your closest relationship where you want it to be?
- ☐ Yes
- ☐ No (10 points)
- ☐ Working on it (5 points)

Are you happy?
- ☐ Yes, generally
- ☐ Some of the time (5 points)
- ☐ Only occasionally (10 points)

Do you have your values written down?
- ☐ Yes
- ☐ No (10 points)

Do you love yourself?
- ☐ Yes (minus 10 points)
- ☐ Maybe (0 points)
- ☐ No (10 points)

TOTAL YOUR POINTS = _____ ON DATE: _____

Low Priority   Under 50

Medium Priority   50-150

High Priority   Over 150

RE-ASSESS AFTER 12 WEEKS

TOTAL YOUR POINTS = _____ ON DATE: _____

APPENDIX III
12 WEEK
"INCH LOSS"
PROGRAMME

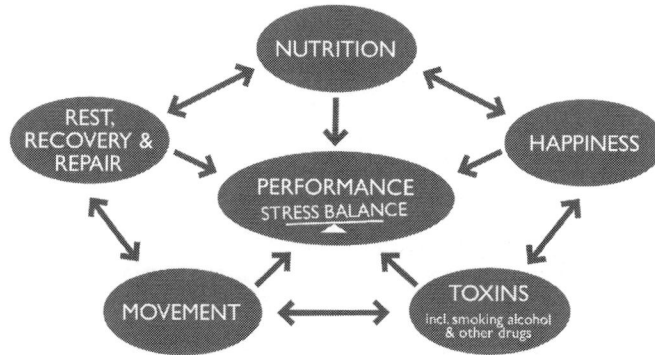

1   REST, RECOVERY & REPAIR

Recovery is often overlooked. But, as any Olympic athlete will tell you, this is what creates the Gold Medal performance. Cellular regeneration has been shown to be key for health. Regeneration will be most effective when the body is in a state of recovery.

2   MOVEMENT

The body requires movement to assist the heart with circulation. The heart is the size of a fist and pumps 7200 litres/day of blood for a lifetime with no annual service – so it needs looking after!

The latest research and epidemiological studies suggest that a different approach to movement than the one recommended at the moment would produce better results. The two main components of this new approach are:

- **NEAT** – **N**on **E**xercise **A**ctivity **T**hermogenesis (increasing low intensity everyday movement)
- **HIT** – **H**igh **I**ntensity **T**raining

3   NUTRITION

ONE MAN'S FOOD IS ANOTHER MAN'S POISON

Firstly, each individual is biochemically unique. This means that the same food may have opposing energetic effects on two different people. Individuals need to understand their own unique metabolism and personalise their diet accordingly.

Secondly, not all calories are equal. For optimal performance the three key nutritional concerns are QUALITY, QUALITY and QUALITY.

4   TOXINS

Out of the five areas, toxins are the biggest user of energy, depleting the functional reserve the most. Our evolutionary body was not designed to deal with the modern toxins it comes into contact with in the 21st century.

Toxic synthetic chemicals are highly fat soluble. When exposed to toxins, the body creates fat to safely store the ones it cannot process and eliminate safely. This is why the world population is getting fatter......

- *1 billion overweight adults in the world. Some 300 million are obese.*
- *One in four adults is currently obese and nine in 10 will be overweight or obese by 2050.*

Therefore the body's exposure to toxins should be reduced as much as possible.

5   HAPPINESS

Governments and businesses alike are beginning to understand that happiness is an important part of an individual or company performance. Those that enjoy what they do, do it better. Happy people are more sociable, flexible, creative and are able to tolerate life's daily frustrations.

Individuals have a choice on whether to be happy or unhappy.

"OTHER PEOPLE CAN NEITHER MAKE US MISERABLE OR HAPPY, ALL WE CAN GET FROM THEM IS INFORMATION, WE DECIDE WHAT TO DO WITH THIS INFORMATION."

GLASSER

Strategies to help individuals choose to enjoy what they do, include looking at individuals' core values.

ENERGY BALANCE AUDIT

AUDIT YOUR LIFE BY WRITING DOWN YOUR ENERGY BUILDING AND YOUR ENERGY DEPLETING ACTIVITIES/BEHAVIOURS

ENERGY BUILDING

Parasympathic PNS (rest/repair)
Anabolic
Ying

ENERGY BALANCE AUDIT

ENERGY DEPLETING

Sympathetic SNS (fight/flight)
Catabolic
Yang

THE LAW OF ATTRACTION

– YOU INEVITABLY ATTRACT INTO YOUR LIFE THE PEOPLE, CIRCUMSTANCE, IDEAS AND RESOURCES IN HARMONY WITH YOU DOMINANT THOUGHTS.

MY DREAM IS?

_____
_____
_____
_____
_____
_____
_____

VALUES

My physical health needs are:

_____
_____
_____
_____

My mental health needs are:

_____
_____
_____
_____

My time needs are:

_____
_____
_____
_____

My rhythm is:

_____
_____
_____
_____

My spiritual philosophy is:

_____
_____
_____

My space needs are:

_____
_____
_____
_____

My family needs are:

_____
_____
_____
_____

My cultural needs are:

_____
_____
_____
_____

My social needs are:

_____
_____
_____
_____

This understanding of yourself is a necessary first step in establishing values that are outwardly or otherwise directed. You cannot value others and you cannot give to others until you understand yourself and live by your own values first. This is why you need to start with your own personal values. All of these values give you the energy to have a 'we' (relationship) and 'all' (family/friends) life.

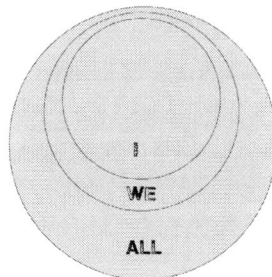

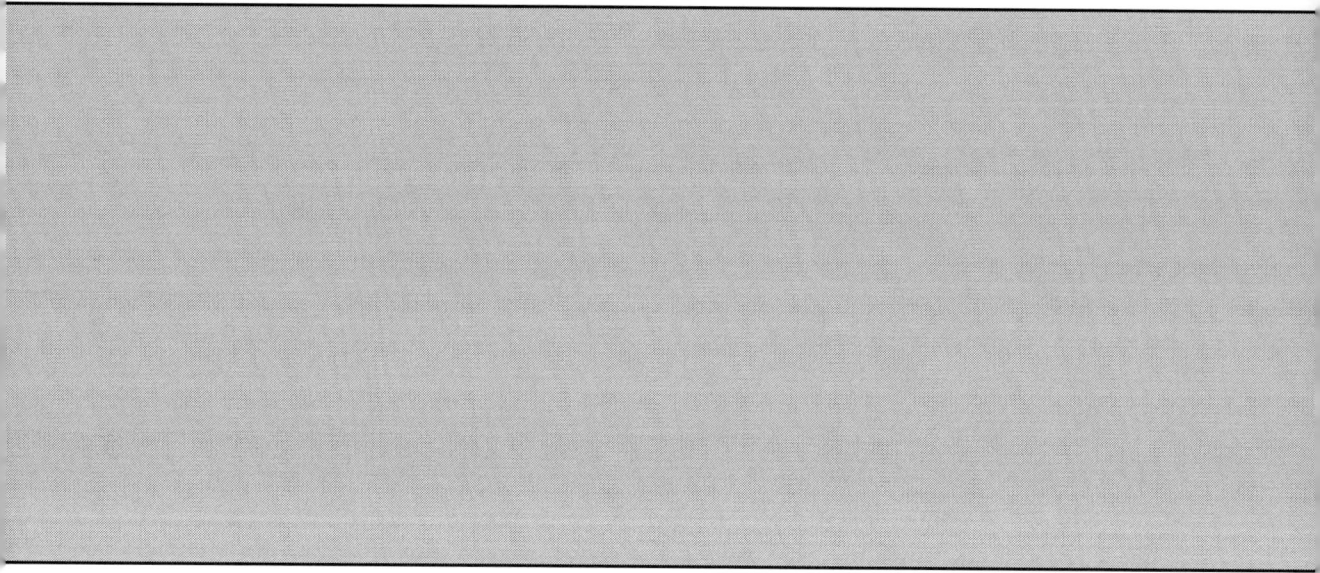

MACRO-NUTRIENTS

Everything you eat or drink falls under the heading of one or more of the three macro-nutrients, which are:

- Protein
- Fat
- Carbohydrate

PROTEINS

MEAT, POULTRY, DAIRY.

The main structural ingredient of human cells and the enzymes that keep them running.

Amino acids are the building blocks of protein

Must get 8 amino acids from diet to enable manufacture of proteins in body

A vegetarian diet does not provide complete proteins and must combine incomplete proteins to enable protein synthesis (dairy, eggs and flesh foods are complete proteins).

Many nutrients better are better absorbed from or in the presence of animal products.

Protein needs to come from high quality sources

FATS

OIL, NUTS, MEAT, CHEESE

Vital structural and functional materials
Concentrated source of energy
Building blocks, especially for cell membranes and hormones
Hormone-like regulating substances (prostaglandins)
Role in absorption of fat-soluble vitamins (A,D,E and K)
Responsible for healthy nerve conduction
Vitamin A & D only found in animal fat.
Cholesterol is an important nutrient (Mother's milk 55% Chol.)
Deficiencies in essentials fatty acids can lead to disease.

ESSENTIAL FATTY ACIDS

Omega 6 & omega 3 must be got from diet
All others can be made from these
Ancestors ate in 50:50 now we eat 3% Omega 3 & 97% Omega 6
Omega 3 sources – fish, raw nuts & seeds
Omega 6 sources – dairy, animal meats, vege, oils

CHEMICALLY ALTERED UNSATURATED FATTY ACIDS

Hydrogenation – alters liquid unsaturated oil into more saturated fat ('cis' to 'trans') – with a longer shelf life
Margarines, salad dressings, baked goods, ice cream, chocolate, snack foods
Potentially carcinogenic, disrupts normal metabolism, interferes with prostaglandin synthesis, banned in many countries!

CARBOHYDRATES

VEGETABLES, FRUITS, GRAINS & BEANS.

Breaks down into starch and sugar.
Principal source of energy for all body functions and structural component of cell walls and plasma membrane.
Vegetables are most nutrient rich 'carbs' - eat lightly cooked (steamed) or raw.
Can be stored in almost unlimited amounts of fat.

USE GLYCEMIC INDEX (GI).

Mostly low – above ground vegetables.
Some medium – fruits, potatoes, carrots.
Few high – bread, rice pasta.

CHOOSE WIDE VARIETY TO GET FIBRE.

Assists digestion, elimination and detoxification.
Lowers blood fats, balances blood sugar, improves energy and immunity, decreases risk of digestive and bowel disorders, even colon cancer.

CAUTION WITH FRUIT

Hybridized for size & sweet taste.
Can lead to carb cravings.
Fruit juice = sugar water (consume small quantities and only freshly squeezed.

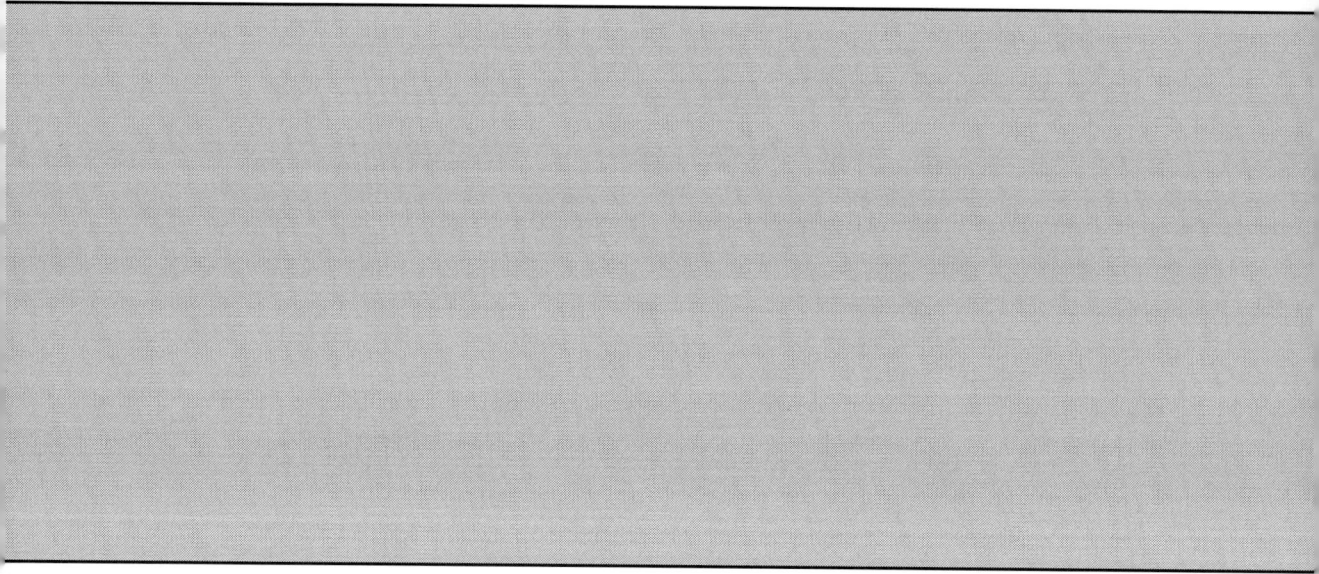

APPENDIX IV
12 WEEK PLAN

WEEK ONE

Movement:	Buy a pedometer & complete 10,000 steps a day
Rest/Repair:	Go to bed/sleep by 10:30pm
Diet:	Only eat real, unprocessed (unpackaged) food
De-tox:	Drink purified water (your bodyweight in kg's x 0.033 = litres)
Happiness:	Think about and write down your dream/legacy

WEEK TWO

Movement:	Become an exercise opportunist
Rest/Repair:	Relax after 9pm without any stimulants eg TV, computer etc
Diet:	Eat more protein & fat
De-tox:	Read labels on everything that goes in or on your body
Happiness:	Start a daily Food & Lifestyle dairy

WEEK THREE

Movement:	20 minutes movement outside a day (in winter between 12-3pm)
Rest/Repair:	10 diaphragm breaths a couple of times everyday this week
Diet:	Remove grains from your diet especially gluten (bread, pasta, flour etc)
De-tox:	Only use organic & natural skin care, cosmetics & haircare
Happiness:	Write down your values & make a daily/weekly plan

WEEK FOUR

Movement:	Have your posture assessed and start a corrective exercise programme
Rest/Repair:	Look at your energy building list and try one of these
Diet:	Quality over quantity – organic, free range, home grown, butchers
De-tox:	If you can't pronounce the word on the label do not eat it
Happiness:	Become aware of your thoughts and turn all negative thoughts into positive ones

WEEK FIVE

Movement:	Try a new movement activity ideally fun & outside
Rest/Repair:	Assess the quality of your sleep this week (use Food Lifestyle Diary)
Diet:	Eat every 4 hours a mix of carbs/fat/protein
De-tox:	Remove ELM from bedroom
Happiness:	Spend some time in nature & laugh out loud each day

WEEK SIX

Movement:	Sign up to a movement challenge (possibly connected to new activity)
Rest/Repair:	Try a meditation CD
Diet:	Take a basic metabolic typing test to personalise your diet
De-tox:	Store mobile phone away from body (not in your pocket for long periods)
Happiness:	Look in mirror and tell yourself you love yourself five times

WEEK SEVEN

Movement:	If you're not still doing the new movement activity try a new
Rest/Repair:	Walk barefoot outside in the bright daylight/sunshine
Diet:	Focus on reactions after food this week (use Food Lifestyle Diary)
De-tox:	Walk barefoot outside in the bright daylight/sunshine
Happiness:	Be thankful for all the things you normally take for granted this week

WEEK EIGHT

Movement:	Try minimalist or barefoot shoes (eg. Vibram Fivefingers) for movement sessions (including running)
Rest/Repair:	20 minutes 2x/wk Meditation/Yoga/Tai Chi/CHEK Zone etc
Diet:	Remove dairy (apart from butter) from your diet for 2 weeks
De-tox:	Avoid plastics, foil, clingfilm etc in food preparation
Happiness:	Create a ritual (such as in the shower each morning) to appreciate your body each day

WEEK NINE

Movement:	Try some HIT training eg 5 x 15secs bursts of 100% effort 2 or 3 times this week
Rest/Repair:	20 minutes 3x/wk Meditation/Yoga/Tai Chi/CHEK Zone etc
Diet:	Avoid so-called health products anything 'low-fat', 'no sugar', 'diet', 'lo cal', soya, 'healthy range', calories written on packaging
De-tox:	Alternate hot/cold in the shower (or sauna & cold plunge)
Happiness:	Think of someone who has wronged you, understand that they (like you) are doing their best from their state of consciousness and then forgive them (you do this for your sake not theirs)

WEEK TEN

Movement:	Two low intensity longer workouts & 2 short high intensity
Rest/Repair:	20 minutes 4x/wk Meditation/Yoga/Tai Chi/CHEK Zone etc
Diet:	After 2 weeks try some dairy and monitor reactions (can do same for gluten)
De-tox:	Assess the quality of the air you breathe and consider some house/office plants
Happiness:	Plan something really fun this week

WEEK ELEVEN

Movement:	Two low intensity longer workouts & 2 short high intensity
Rest/Repair:	20 minutes 5x/wk Meditation/Yoga/Tai Chi/CHEK Zone etc
Diet:	If it wasn't around 10,000 years ago don't eat it
De-tox:	Limit time on electrical devices
Happiness:	Be aware of your energy and how to build and protect it, who builds energy and who depletes your energy levels

WEEK TWELVE

Movement:	Two low intensity longer workouts & 2 short high intensity
Rest/Repair:	20 minutes 6x/wk Meditation/Yoga/Tai Chi/CHEK Zone etc
Diet:	Use 80:20 rule eat right 80% of time, you can do what you want 20% of the time
De-tox:	Improve liver function by eating dark green leafy vegetables, garlic, onions, cabbage, broccoli, milk thistle
Happiness:	Love in action can only produce happiness – practise love

TUMMY MEASUREMENTS

FORGET WEIGHT, THROW AWAY THOSE SCALES, AND MEASURE AROUND YOUR TUMMY INSTEAD.

OVER 100CM = "SERIOUS HEALTH RISK"

MEASUREMENT AROUND MIDDLE AT LEVEL OF TUMMY BUTTON

Week 0	_____ cm
Week 1	_____ cm
Week 2	_____ cm
Week 3	_____ cm
Week 4	_____ cm
Week 5	_____ cm
Week 6	_____ cm
Week 7	_____ cm
Week 8	_____ cm
Week 9	_____ cm
Week 10	_____ cm
Week 11	_____ cm
Week 12	_____ cm

Notes: same time each week

DAILY FOOD & LIFESTYLE DIARY

DAILY FOOD DIARY - DATE: _____

Complete everyday for 12 weeks

MEAL 1 – TIME: _____

Please fill out form 1-2 hours after each meal

Most likely too many carbs	Balanced Responses	Most likely too much protein &/or fat	
☐ Headache	☐ Appetite feels satisfied	☐ Lethargic	Approx. of macro Nutrient ratios of meal
☐ Anxiety	☐ Feel emotionally balanced	☐ Mentally Sluggish	% Carbs _____
☐ Jittery/wired	☐ Good mental focus	☐ Heavy Gut	% Protein _____
☐ Difficulty concentrating	☐ Normal level of energy	☐ Feel full yet still hungry	% Fat _____
☐ Hunger is not satisfied	☐ No cravings for sweets	☐ Crave sweets	Foods Eaten: _____
☐ Crave sweet	☐ No cravings for more food	☐ Crave Caffeine	_____
☐ Crave Protein & fat		(if more than hour after meal could	_____
		be a crash from too much carb)	_____

MEAL 2 – TIME: _____

Most likely too many carbs	Balanced Responses	Most likely too much protein &/or fat	
☐ Headache	☐ Appetite feels satisfied	☐ Lethargic	Approx. of macro Nutrient ratios of meal
☐ Anxiety	☐ Feel emotionally balanced	☐ Mentally Sluggish	% Carbs _____
☐ Jittery/wired	☐ Good mental focus	☐ Heavy Gut	% Protein _____
☐ Difficulty concentrating	☐ Normal level of energy	☐ Feel full yet still hungry	% Fat _____
☐ Hunger is not satisfied	☐ No cravings for sweets	☐ Crave sweets	Foods Eaten: _____
☐ Crave sweet	☐ No cravings for more food	☐ Crave Caffeine	_____
☐ Crave Protein & fat		(if more than hour after meal could	_____
		be a crash from too much carb)	_____

MEAL 3 – TIME: _____

Most likely too many carbs	Balanced Responses	Most likely too much protein &/or fat	
☐ Headache	☐ Appetite feels satisfied	☐ Lethargic	Approx. of macro Nutrient ratios of meal
☐ Anxiety	☐ Feel emotionally balanced	☐ Mentally Sluggish	% Carbs _____
☐ Jittery/wired	☐ Good mental focus	☐ Heavy Gut	% Protein _____
☐ Difficulty concentrating	☐ Normal level of energy	☐ Feel full yet still hungry	% Fat _____
☐ Hunger is not satisfied	☐ No cravings for sweets	☐ Crave sweets	Foods Eaten: _____
☐ Crave sweet	☐ No cravings for more food	☐ Crave Caffeine	_____
☐ Crave Protein & fat		(if more than hour after meal could	_____
		be a crash from too much carb)	_____

SNACKS:

Time: _____ Details: _____
Time: _____ Details: _____
Time: _____ Details: _____

DRINKS:

Details: _____
_____
_____

LIFESTYLE:

What time did you go to sleep? _____   What time did you get up? _____   Bowel movement(s)?
Sleep quality? ☐ Sound ☐ Restless   Did you have night Sweats? ☐ Yes ☐ No   (number, colour, size & shape)
Did you awake during night (give time & reason)? _____
Did you wake up refreshed today or tired? ☐ Refreshed ☐ Tired
Did you start slow this morning? ☐ Yes ☐ No   If yes, how long did it take to feel alert? _____

MOVEMENT :

Details: _____
_____

GENERAL:

How did you feel today? _____
_____

OTHER INFO: _____

DAILY FOOD & LIFESTYLE DIARY

DAILY FOOD DIARY - DATE: _____

Complete everyday for 12 weeks

MEAL 1 – TIME: _____

Please fill out form 1-2 hours after each meal

Most likely too many carbs	Balanced Responses	Most likely too much protein &/or fat
☐ Headache	☐ Appetite feels satisfied	☐ Lethargic
☐ Anxiety	☐ Feel emotionally balanced	☐ Mentally Sluggish
☐ Jittery/wired	☐ Good mental focus	☐ Heavy Gut
☐ Difficulty concentrating	☐ Normal level of energy	☐ Feel full yet still hungry
☐ Hunger is not satisfied	☐ No cravings for sweets	☐ Crave sweets
☐ Crave sweet	☐ No cravings for more food	☐ Crave Caffeine
☐ Crave Protein & fat		(if more than hour after meal could be a crash from too much carb)

Approx. of macro Nutrient ratios of meal
% Carbs _____
% Protein _____
% Fat _____
Foods Eaten: _____
_____
_____
_____
_____

MEAL 2 – TIME: _____

Most likely too many carbs	Balanced Responses	Most likely too much protein &/or fat
☐ Headache	☐ Appetite feels satisfied	☐ Lethargic
☐ Anxiety	☐ Feel emotionally balanced	☐ Mentally Sluggish
☐ Jittery/wired	☐ Good mental focus	☐ Heavy Gut
☐ Difficulty concentrating	☐ Normal level of energy	☐ Feel full yet still hungry
☐ Hunger is not satisfied	☐ No cravings for sweets	☐ Crave sweets
☐ Crave sweet	☐ No cravings for more food	☐ Crave Caffeine
☐ Crave Protein & fat		(if more than hour after meal could be a crash from too much carb)

Approx. of macro Nutrient ratios of meal
% Carbs _____
% Protein _____
% Fat _____
Foods Eaten: _____
_____
_____
_____
_____

MEAL 3 – TIME: _____

Most likely too many carbs	Balanced Responses	Most likely too much protein &/or fat
☐ Headache	☐ Appetite feels satisfied	☐ Lethargic
☐ Anxiety	☐ Feel emotionally balanced	☐ Mentally Sluggish
☐ Jittery/wired	☐ Good mental focus	☐ Heavy Gut
☐ Difficulty concentrating	☐ Normal level of energy	☐ Feel full yet still hungry
☐ Hunger is not satisfied	☐ No cravings for sweets	☐ Crave sweets
☐ Crave sweet	☐ No cravings for more food	☐ Crave Caffeine
☐ Crave Protein & fat		(if more than hour after meal could be a crash from too much carb)

Approx. of macro Nutrient ratios of meal
% Carbs _____
% Protein _____
% Fat _____
Foods Eaten: _____
_____
_____
_____
_____

SNACKS:

Time: _____ Details: _____
Time: _____ Details: _____
Time: _____ Details: _____

DRINKS:

Details: _____
_____
_____

LIFESTYLE:

What time did you go to sleep? _____   What time did you get up? _____
Sleep quality? ☐ Sound ☐ Restless   Did you have night Sweats? ☐ Yes ☐ No
Did you awake during night (give time & reason)? _____
Did you wake up refreshed today or tired? ☐ Refreshed ☐ Tired
Did you start slow this morning? ☐ Yes ☐ No   If yes, how long did it take to feel alert? _____

Bowel movement(s)?
(number, colour, size & shape)
_____
_____

MOVEMENT :

Details: _____
_____
_____

GENERAL:

How did you feel today? _____
_____
_____

OTHER INFO: _____

DAILY FOOD & LIFESTYLE DIARY

DAILY FOOD DIARY - DATE: _____

Complete everyday for 12 weeks

MEAL 1 – TIME: _____

Please fill out form 1-2 hours after each meal

Most likely too many carbs	Balanced Responses	Most likely too much protein &/or fat	
☐ Headache	☐ Appetite feels satisfied	☐ Lethargic	Approx. of macro Nutrient ratios of meal
☐ Anxiety	☐ Feel emotionally balanced	☐ Mentally Sluggish	% Carbs _____
☐ Jittery/wired	☐ Good mental focus	☐ Heavy Gut	% Protein _____
☐ Difficulty concentrating	☐ Normal level of energy	☐ Feel full yet still hungry	% Fat _____
☐ Hunger is not satisfied	☐ No cravings for sweets	☐ Crave sweets	Foods Eaten: _____
☐ Crave sweet	☐ No cravings for more food	☐ Crave Caffeine	_____
☐ Crave Protein & fat		(if more than hour after meal could	_____
		be a crash from too much carb)	_____
			_____
			_____

MEAL 2 – TIME: _____

Most likely too many carbs	Balanced Responses	Most likely too much protein &/or fat	
☐ Headache	☐ Appetite feels satisfied	☐ Lethargic	Approx. of macro Nutrient ratios of meal
☐ Anxiety	☐ Feel emotionally balanced	☐ Mentally Sluggish	% Carbs _____
☐ Jittery/wired	☐ Good mental focus	☐ Heavy Gut	% Protein _____
☐ Difficulty concentrating	☐ Normal level of energy	☐ Feel full yet still hungry	% Fat _____
☐ Hunger is not satisfied	☐ No cravings for sweets	☐ Crave sweets	Foods Eaten: _____
☐ Crave sweet	☐ No cravings for more food	☐ Crave Caffeine	_____
☐ Crave Protein & fat		(if more than hour after meal could	_____
		be a crash from too much carb)	_____
			_____
			_____

MEAL 3 – TIME: _____

Most likely too many carbs	Balanced Responses	Most likely too much protein &/or fat	
☐ Headache	☐ Appetite feels satisfied	☐ Lethargic	Approx. of macro Nutrient ratios of meal
☐ Anxiety	☐ Feel emotionally balanced	☐ Mentally Sluggish	% Carbs _____
☐ Jittery/wired	☐ Good mental focus	☐ Heavy Gut	% Protein _____
☐ Difficulty concentrating	☐ Normal level of energy	☐ Feel full yet still hungry	% Fat _____
☐ Hunger is not satisfied	☐ No cravings for sweets	☐ Crave sweets	Foods Eaten: _____
☐ Crave sweet	☐ No cravings for more food	☐ Crave Caffeine	_____
☐ Crave Protein & fat		(if more than hour after meal could	_____
		be a crash from too much carb)	_____
			_____
			_____

SNACKS:

Time: _____ Details: _____

Time: _____ Details: _____

Time: _____ Details: _____

DRINKS:

Details: _____

_____

_____

LIFESTYLE:

What time did you go to sleep? _____ What time did you get up? _____

Sleep quality? ☐ Sound ☐ Restless   Did you have night Sweats? ☐ Yes ☐ No

Did you awake during night (give time & reason)? _____

Did you wake up refreshed today or tired? ☐ Refreshed ☐ Tired

Did you start slow this morning? ☐ Yes ☐ No   If yes, how long did it take to feel alert? _____

Bowel movement(s)?
(number, colour, size & shape)

_____

_____

MOVEMENT :

Details: _____

_____

_____

GENERAL:

How did you feel today? _____

_____

_____

OTHER INFO: _____

DAILY FOOD & LIFESTYLE DIARY

DAILY FOOD DIARY - DATE: _____   Complete everyday for 12 weeks

MEAL 1 – TIME: _____   Please fill out form 1-2 hours after each meal

Most likely too many carbs	Balanced Responses	Most likely too much protein &/or fat	
☐ Headache	☐ Appetite feels satisfied	☐ Lethargic	Approx. of macro Nutrient ratios of meal
☐ Anxiety	☐ Feel emotionally balanced	☐ Mentally Sluggish	% Carbs _____
☐ Jittery/wired	☐ Good mental focus	☐ Heavy Gut	% Protein _____
☐ Difficulty concentrating	☐ Normal level of energy	☐ Feel full yet still hungry	% Fat _____
☐ Hunger is not satisfied	☐ No cravings for sweets	☐ Crave sweets	Foods Eaten: _____
☐ Crave sweet	☐ No cravings for more food	☐ Crave Caffeine	_____
☐ Crave Protein & fat		(if more than hour after meal could	_____
		be a crash from too much carb)	_____

MEAL 2 – TIME: _____

Most likely too many carbs	Balanced Responses	Most likely too much protein &/or fat	
☐ Headache	☐ Appetite feels satisfied	☐ Lethargic	Approx. of macro Nutrient ratios of meal
☐ Anxiety	☐ Feel emotionally balanced	☐ Mentally Sluggish	% Carbs _____
☐ Jittery/wired	☐ Good mental focus	☐ Heavy Gut	% Protein _____
☐ Difficulty concentrating	☐ Normal level of energy	☐ Feel full yet still hungry	% Fat _____
☐ Hunger is not satisfied	☐ No cravings for sweets	☐ Crave sweets	Foods Eaten: _____
☐ Crave sweet	☐ No cravings for more food	☐ Crave Caffeine	_____
☐ Crave Protein & fat		(if more than hour after meal could	_____
		be a crash from too much carb)	_____

MEAL 3 – TIME: _____

Most likely too many carbs	Balanced Responses	Most likely too much protein &/or fat	
☐ Headache	☐ Appetite feels satisfied	☐ Lethargic	Approx. of macro Nutrient ratios of meal
☐ Anxiety	☐ Feel emotionally balanced	☐ Mentally Sluggish	% Carbs _____
☐ Jittery/wired	☐ Good mental focus	☐ Heavy Gut	% Protein _____
☐ Difficulty concentrating	☐ Normal level of energy	☐ Feel full yet still hungry	% Fat _____
☐ Hunger is not satisfied	☐ No cravings for sweets	☐ Crave sweets	Foods Eaten: _____
☐ Crave sweet	☐ No cravings for more food	☐ Crave Caffeine	_____
☐ Crave Protein & fat		(if more than hour after meal could	_____
		be a crash from too much carb)	_____

SNACKS:

Time: _____ Details: _____

Time: _____ Details: _____

Time: _____ Details: _____

DRINKS:

Details: _____

_____

_____

LIFESTYLE:

What time did you go to sleep? _____ What time did you get up? _____

Sleep quality? ☐ Sound ☐ Restless   Did you have night Sweats? ☐ Yes ☐ No

Did you awake during night (give time & reason)? _____

Did you wake up refreshed today or tired? ☐ Refreshed ☐ Tired

Did you start slow this morning? ☐ Yes ☐ No   If yes, how long did it take to feel alert? _____

Bowel movement(s)?
(number, colour, size & shape)

_____

_____

MOVEMENT :

Details: _____

_____

_____

GENERAL:

How did you feel today? _____

_____

OTHER INFO: _____

DAILY FOOD & LIFESTYLE DIARY

DAILY FOOD DIARY - DATE: _____   Complete everyday for 12 weeks

MEAL 1 – TIME: _____   Please fill out form 1-2 hours after each meal

Most likely too many carbs	Balanced Responses	Most likely too much protein &/or fat	
☐ Headache	☐ Appetite feels satisfied	☐ Lethargic	Approx. of macro Nutrient ratios of meal
☐ Anxiety	☐ Feel emotionally balanced	☐ Mentally Sluggish	% Carbs _____
☐ Jittery/wired	☐ Good mental focus	☐ Heavy Gut	% Protein _____
☐ Difficulty concentrating	☐ Normal level of energy	☐ Feel full yet still hungry	% Fat _____
☐ Hunger is not satisfied	☐ No cravings for sweets	☐ Crave sweets	Foods Eaten: _____
☐ Crave sweet	☐ No cravings for more food	☐ Crave Caffeine	_____
☐ Crave Protein & fat		(if more than hour after meal could	_____
		be a crash from too much carb)	_____
			_____
			_____

MEAL 2 – TIME: _____

Most likely too many carbs	Balanced Responses	Most likely too much protein &/or fat	
☐ Headache	☐ Appetite feels satisfied	☐ Lethargic	Approx. of macro Nutrient ratios of meal
☐ Anxiety	☐ Feel emotionally balanced	☐ Mentally Sluggish	% Carbs _____
☐ Jittery/wired	☐ Good mental focus	☐ Heavy Gut	% Protein _____
☐ Difficulty concentrating	☐ Normal level of energy	☐ Feel full yet still hungry	% Fat _____
☐ Hunger is not satisfied	☐ No cravings for sweets	☐ Crave sweets	Foods Eaten: _____
☐ Crave sweet	☐ No cravings for more food	☐ Crave Caffeine	_____
☐ Crave Protein & fat		(if more than hour after meal could	_____
		be a crash from too much carb)	_____
			_____
			_____

MEAL 3 – TIME: _____

Most likely too many carbs	Balanced Responses	Most likely too much protein &/or fat	
☐ Headache	☐ Appetite feels satisfied	☐ Lethargic	Approx. of macro Nutrient ratios of meal
☐ Anxiety	☐ Feel emotionally balanced	☐ Mentally Sluggish	% Carbs _____
☐ Jittery/wired	☐ Good mental focus	☐ Heavy Gut	% Protein _____
☐ Difficulty concentrating	☐ Normal level of energy	☐ Feel full yet still hungry	% Fat _____
☐ Hunger is not satisfied	☐ No cravings for sweets	☐ Crave sweets	Foods Eaten: _____
☐ Crave sweet	☐ No cravings for more food	☐ Crave Caffeine	_____
☐ Crave Protein & fat		(if more than hour after meal could	_____
		be a crash from too much carb)	_____
			_____
			_____

SNACKS: **DRINKS:**

Time: _____ Details: _____   Details: _____

Time: _____ Details: _____   _____

Time: _____ Details: _____   _____

LIFESTYLE:

What time did you go to sleep?_____   What time did you get up? _____   Bowel movement(s)?

Sleep quality? ☐ Sound ☐ Restless   Did you have night Sweats? ☐ Yes ☐ No   (number, colour, size & shape)

Did you awake during night (give time & reason)? _____

Did you wake up refreshed today or tired? ☐ Refreshed ☐ Tired   _____

Did you start slow this morning? ☐ Yes ☐ No   If yes, how long did it take to feel alert? _____

MOVEMENT :   **GENERAL:**

Details: _____   How did you feel today? _____

_____   _____

_____   _____

OTHER INFO: _____

DAILY FOOD & LIFESTYLE DIARY

DAILY FOOD DIARY - DATE: _____   Complete everyday for 12 weeks

MEAL 1 – TIME: _____   Please fill out form 1-2 hours after each meal

Most likely too many carbs	Balanced Responses	Most likely too much protein &/or fat	
☐ Headache	☐ Appetite feels satisfied	☐ Lethargic	Approx. of macro Nutrient ratios of meal
☐ Anxiety	☐ Feel emotionally balanced	☐ Mentally Sluggish	% Carbs _____
☐ Jittery/wired	☐ Good mental focus	☐ Heavy Gut	% Protein _____
☐ Difficulty concentrating	☐ Normal level of energy	☐ Feel full yet still hungry	% Fat _____
☐ Hunger is not satisfied	☐ No cravings for sweets	☐ Crave sweets	Foods Eaten: _____
☐ Crave sweet	☐ No cravings for more food	☐ Crave Caffeine	_____
☐ Crave Protein & fat		(if more than hour after meal could	_____
		be a crash from too much carb)	_____

MEAL 2 – TIME: _____

Most likely too many carbs	Balanced Responses	Most likely too much protein &/or fat	
☐ Headache	☐ Appetite feels satisfied	☐ Lethargic	Approx. of macro Nutrient ratios of meal
☐ Anxiety	☐ Feel emotionally balanced	☐ Mentally Sluggish	% Carbs _____
☐ Jittery/wired	☐ Good mental focus	☐ Heavy Gut	% Protein _____
☐ Difficulty concentrating	☐ Normal level of energy	☐ Feel full yet still hungry	% Fat _____
☐ Hunger is not satisfied	☐ No cravings for sweets	☐ Crave sweets	Foods Eaten: _____
☐ Crave sweet	☐ No cravings for more food	☐ Crave Caffeine	_____
☐ Crave Protein & fat		(if more than hour after meal could	_____
		be a crash from too much carb)	_____

MEAL 3 – TIME: _____

Most likely too many carbs	Balanced Responses	Most likely too much protein &/or fat	
☐ Headache	☐ Appetite feels satisfied	☐ Lethargic	Approx. of macro Nutrient ratios of meal
☐ Anxiety	☐ Feel emotionally balanced	☐ Mentally Sluggish	% Carbs _____
☐ Jittery/wired	☐ Good mental focus	☐ Heavy Gut	% Protein _____
☐ Difficulty concentrating	☐ Normal level of energy	☐ Feel full yet still hungry	% Fat _____
☐ Hunger is not satisfied	☐ No cravings for sweets	☐ Crave sweets	Foods Eaten: _____
☐ Crave sweet	☐ No cravings for more food	☐ Crave Caffeine	_____
☐ Crave Protein & fat		(if more than hour after meal could	_____
		be a crash from too much carb)	_____

SNACKS: **DRINKS:**

Time: _____ Details: _____   Details: _____

Time: _____ Details: _____   _____

Time: _____ Details: _____   _____

LIFESTYLE:

What time did you go to sleep?_____   What time did you get up? _____   Bowel movement(s)?

Sleep quality? ☐ Sound ☐ Restless   Did you have night Sweats? ☐ Yes ☐ No   (number, colour, size & shape)

Did you awake during night (give time & reason)? _____   _____

Did you wake up refreshed today or tired? ☐ Refreshed ☐ Tired   _____

Did you start slow this morning? ☐ Yes ☐ No   If yes, how long did it take to feel alert? _____

MOVEMENT :   **GENERAL:**

Details: _____   How did you feel today? _____

_____   _____

OTHER INFO: _____

DAILY FOOD & LIFESTYLE DIARY

DAILY FOOD DIARY - DATE: _____

Complete everyday for 12 weeks

MEAL 1 – TIME: _____

Please fill out form 1-2 hours after each meal

Most likely too many carbs	Balanced Responses	Most likely too much protein &/or fat	
☐ Headache	☐ Appetite feels satisfied	☐ Lethargic	Approx. of macro Nutrient ratios of meal
☐ Anxiety	☐ Feel emotionally balanced	☐ Mentally Sluggish	% Carbs _____
☐ Jittery/wired	☐ Good mental focus	☐ Heavy Gut	% Protein _____
☐ Difficulty concentrating	☐ Normal level of energy	☐ Feel full yet still hungry	% Fat _____
☐ Hunger is not satisfied	☐ No cravings for sweets	☐ Crave sweets	Foods Eaten: _____
☐ Crave sweet	☐ No cravings for more food	☐ Crave Caffeine	_____
☐ Crave Protein & fat		(if more than hour after meal could	_____
		be a crash from too much carb)	_____

MEAL 2 – TIME: _____

Most likely too many carbs	Balanced Responses	Most likely too much protein &/or fat	
☐ Headache	☐ Appetite feels satisfied	☐ Lethargic	Approx. of macro Nutrient ratios of meal
☐ Anxiety	☐ Feel emotionally balanced	☐ Mentally Sluggish	% Carbs _____
☐ Jittery/wired	☐ Good mental focus	☐ Heavy Gut	% Protein _____
☐ Difficulty concentrating	☐ Normal level of energy	☐ Feel full yet still hungry	% Fat _____
☐ Hunger is not satisfied	☐ No cravings for sweets	☐ Crave sweets	Foods Eaten: _____
☐ Crave sweet	☐ No cravings for more food	☐ Crave Caffeine	_____
☐ Crave Protein & fat		(if more than hour after meal could	_____
		be a crash from too much carb)	_____

MEAL 3 – TIME: _____

Most likely too many carbs	Balanced Responses	Most likely too much protein &/or fat	
☐ Headache	☐ Appetite feels satisfied	☐ Lethargic	Approx. of macro Nutrient ratios of meal
☐ Anxiety	☐ Feel emotionally balanced	☐ Mentally Sluggish	% Carbs _____
☐ Jittery/wired	☐ Good mental focus	☐ Heavy Gut	% Protein _____
☐ Difficulty concentrating	☐ Normal level of energy	☐ Feel full yet still hungry	% Fat _____
☐ Hunger is not satisfied	☐ No cravings for sweets	☐ Crave sweets	Foods Eaten: _____
☐ Crave sweet	☐ No cravings for more food	☐ Crave Caffeine	_____
☐ Crave Protein & fat		(if more than hour after meal could	_____
		be a crash from too much carb)	_____

SNACKS:

Time: _____ Details: _____

Time: _____ Details: _____

Time: _____ Details: _____

DRINKS:

Details: _____

_____

_____

LIFESTYLE:

What time did you go to sleep?_____ What time did you get up? _____ Bowel movement(s)?

Sleep quality? ☐ Sound ☐ Restless   Did you have night Sweats? ☐ Yes ☐ No   (number, colour, size & shape)

Did you awake during night (give time & reason)? _____

Did you wake up refreshed today or tired? ☐ Refreshed ☐ Tired

Did you start slow this morning? ☐ Yes ☐ No   If yes, how long did it take to feel alert? _____

MOVEMENT :

Details:_____

_____

_____

GENERAL:

How did you feel today? _____

_____

OTHER INFO: _____

DAILY FOOD & LIFESTYLE DIARY

DAILY FOOD DIARY - DATE: _____

MEAL 1 – TIME: _____

Complete everyday for 12 weeks

Please fill out form 1-2 hours after each meal

Most likely too many carbs	Balanced Responses
☐ Headache	☐ Appetite feels satisfied
☐ Anxiety	☐ Feel emotionally balanced
☐ Jittery/wired	☐ Good mental focus
☐ Difficulty concentrating	☐ Normal level of energy
☐ Hunger is not satisfied	☐ No cravings for sweets
☐ Crave sweet	☐ No cravings for more food
☐ Crave Protein & fat	

Most likely too much protein &/or fat

☐ Lethargic
☐ Mentally Sluggish
☐ Heavy Gut
☐ Feel full yet still hungry
☐ Crave sweets
☐ Crave Caffeine
(if more than hour after meal could be a crash from too much carb)

Approx. of macro Nutrient ratios of meal
% Carbs _____
% Protein _____
% Fat _____
Foods Eaten: _____
_____
_____
_____
_____

MEAL 2 – TIME: _____

Most likely too many carbs	Balanced Responses
☐ Headache	☐ Appetite feels satisfied
☐ Anxiety	☐ Feel emotionally balanced
☐ Jittery/wired	☐ Good mental focus
☐ Difficulty concentrating	☐ Normal level of energy
☐ Hunger is not satisfied	☐ No cravings for sweets
☐ Crave sweet	☐ No cravings for more food
☐ Crave Protein & fat	

Most likely too much protein &/or fat

☐ Lethargic
☐ Mentally Sluggish
☐ Heavy Gut
☐ Feel full yet still hungry
☐ Crave sweets
☐ Crave Caffeine
(if more than hour after meal could be a crash from too much carb)

Approx. of macro Nutrient ratios of meal
% Carbs _____
% Protein _____
% Fat _____
Foods Eaten: _____
_____
_____
_____
_____

MEAL 3 – TIME: _____

Most likely too many carbs	Balanced Responses
☐ Headache	☐ Appetite feels satisfied
☐ Anxiety	☐ Feel emotionally balanced
☐ Jittery/wired	☐ Good mental focus
☐ Difficulty concentrating	☐ Normal level of energy
☐ Hunger is not satisfied	☐ No cravings for sweets
☐ Crave sweet	☐ No cravings for more food
☐ Crave Protein & fat	

Most likely too much protein &/or fat

☐ Lethargic
☐ Mentally Sluggish
☐ Heavy Gut
☐ Feel full yet still hungry
☐ Crave sweets
☐ Crave Caffeine
(if more than hour after meal could be a crash from too much carb)

Approx. of macro Nutrient ratios of meal
% Carbs _____
% Protein _____
% Fat _____
Foods Eaten: _____
_____
_____
_____
_____

SNACKS:

Time: _____ Details: _____
Time: _____ Details: _____
Time: _____ Details: _____

DRINKS:

Details: _____
_____
_____

LIFESTYLE:

What time did you go to sleep?_____ What time did you get up? _____
Sleep quality? ☐ Sound ☐ Restless   Did you have night Sweats? ☐ Yes ☐ No
Did you awake during night (give time & reason)? _____
Did you wake up refreshed today or tired? ☐ Refreshed ☐ Tired
Did you start slow this morning? ☐ Yes ☐ No   If yes, how long did it take to feel alert? _____

Bowel movement(s)?
(number, colour, size & shape)
_____
_____

MOVEMENT :

Details: _____
_____
_____

GENERAL:

How did you feel today? _____
_____
_____

OTHER INFO: _____

DAILY FOOD & LIFESTYLE DIARY

DAILY FOOD DIARY - DATE: _____

Complete everyday for 12 weeks

MEAL 1 – TIME: _____

Please fill out form 1-2 hours after each meal

Most likely too many carbs

- ☐ Headache
- ☐ Anxiety
- ☐ Jittery/wired
- ☐ Difficulty concentrating
- ☐ Hunger is not satisfied
- ☐ Crave sweet
- ☐ Crave Protein & fat

Balanced Responses

- ☐ Appetite feels satisfied
- ☐ Feel emotionally balanced
- ☐ Good mental focus
- ☐ Normal level of energy
- ☐ No cravings for sweets
- ☐ No cravings for more food

Most likely too much protein &/or fat

- ☐ Lethargic
- ☐ Mentally Sluggish
- ☐ Heavy Gut
- ☐ Feel full yet still hungry
- ☐ Crave sweets
- ☐ Crave Caffeine

(if more than hour after meal could be a crash from too much carb)

Approx. of macro Nutrient ratios of meal
% Carbs _____
% Protein _____
% Fat _____
Foods Eaten: _____
_____
_____
_____
_____
_____
_____

MEAL 2 – TIME: _____

Most likely too many carbs

- ☐ Headache
- ☐ Anxiety
- ☐ Jittery/wired
- ☐ Difficulty concentrating
- ☐ Hunger is not satisfied
- ☐ Crave sweet
- ☐ Crave Protein & fat

Balanced Responses

- ☐ Appetite feels satisfied
- ☐ Feel emotionally balanced
- ☐ Good mental focus
- ☐ Normal level of energy
- ☐ No cravings for sweets
- ☐ No cravings for more food

Most likely too much protein &/or fat

- ☐ Lethargic
- ☐ Mentally Sluggish
- ☐ Heavy Gut
- ☐ Feel full yet still hungry
- ☐ Crave sweets
- ☐ Crave Caffeine

(if more than hour after meal could be a crash from too much carb)

Approx. of macro Nutrient ratios of meal
% Carbs _____
% Protein _____
% Fat _____
Foods Eaten: _____
_____
_____
_____
_____
_____
_____

MEAL 3 – TIME: _____

Most likely too many carbs

- ☐ Headache
- ☐ Anxiety
- ☐ Jittery/wired
- ☐ Difficulty concentrating
- ☐ Hunger is not satisfied
- ☐ Crave sweet
- ☐ Crave Protein & fat

Balanced Responses

- ☐ Appetite feels satisfied
- ☐ Feel emotionally balanced
- ☐ Good mental focus
- ☐ Normal level of energy
- ☐ No cravings for sweets
- ☐ No cravings for more food

Most likely too much protein &/or fat

- ☐ Lethargic
- ☐ Mentally Sluggish
- ☐ Heavy Gut
- ☐ Feel full yet still hungry
- ☐ Crave sweets
- ☐ Crave Caffeine

(if more than hour after meal could be a crash from too much carb)

Approx. of macro Nutrient ratios of meal
% Carbs _____
% Protein _____
% Fat _____
Foods Eaten: _____
_____
_____
_____
_____
_____

SNACKS:

Time: _____ Details: _____
Time: _____ Details: _____
Time: _____ Details: _____

DRINKS:

Details: _____
_____
_____

LIFESTYLE:

What time did you go to sleep? _____ What time did you get up? _____

Sleep quality? ☐ Sound ☐ Restless   Did you have night Sweats? ☐ Yes ☐ No

Bowel movement(s)?
(number, colour, size & shape)

Did you awake during night (give time & reason)? _____
Did you wake up refreshed today or tired? ☐ Refreshed ☐ Tired
Did you start slow this morning? ☐ Yes ☐ No   If yes, how long did it take to feel alert? _____
_____
_____

MOVEMENT :

Details: _____
_____
_____

GENERAL:

How did you feel today? _____
_____
_____

OTHER INFO: _____

DAILY FOOD & LIFESTYLE DIARY

DAILY FOOD DIARY - DATE: _____

Complete everyday for 12 weeks

MEAL 1 – TIME: _____

Please fill out form 1-2 hours after each meal

Most likely too many carbs	Balanced Responses	Most likely too much protein &/or fat	Approx. of macro Nutrient ratios of meal
☐ Headache	☐ Appetite feels satisfied	☐ Lethargic	% Carbs _____
☐ Anxiety	☐ Feel emotionally balanced	☐ Mentally Sluggish	% Protein _____
☐ Jittery/wired	☐ Good mental focus	☐ Heavy Gut	% Fat _____
☐ Difficulty concentrating	☐ Normal level of energy	☐ Feel full yet still hungry	Foods Eaten: _____
☐ Hunger is not satisfied	☐ No cravings for sweets	☐ Crave sweets	_____
☐ Crave sweet	☐ No cravings for more food	☐ Crave Caffeine	_____
☐ Crave Protein & fat		(if more than hour after meal could be a crash from too much carb)	_____

MEAL 2 – TIME: _____

Most likely too many carbs	Balanced Responses	Most likely too much protein &/or fat	Approx. of macro Nutrient ratios of meal
☐ Headache	☐ Appetite feels satisfied	☐ Lethargic	% Carbs _____
☐ Anxiety	☐ Feel emotionally balanced	☐ Mentally Sluggish	% Protein _____
☐ Jittery/wired	☐ Good mental focus	☐ Heavy Gut	% Fat _____
☐ Difficulty concentrating	☐ Normal level of energy	☐ Feel full yet still hungry	Foods Eaten: _____
☐ Hunger is not satisfied	☐ No cravings for sweets	☐ Crave sweets	_____
☐ Crave sweet	☐ No cravings for more food	☐ Crave Caffeine	_____
☐ Crave Protein & fat		(if more than hour after meal could be a crash from too much carb)	_____

MEAL 3 – TIME: _____

Most likely too many carbs	Balanced Responses	Most likely too much protein &/or fat	Approx. of macro Nutrient ratios of meal
☐ Headache	☐ Appetite feels satisfied	☐ Lethargic	% Carbs _____
☐ Anxiety	☐ Feel emotionally balanced	☐ Mentally Sluggish	% Protein _____
☐ Jittery/wired	☐ Good mental focus	☐ Heavy Gut	% Fat _____
☐ Difficulty concentrating	☐ Normal level of energy	☐ Feel full yet still hungry	Foods Eaten: _____
☐ Hunger is not satisfied	☐ No cravings for sweets	☐ Crave sweets	_____
☐ Crave sweet	☐ No cravings for more food	☐ Crave Caffeine	_____
☐ Crave Protein & fat		(if more than hour after meal could be a crash from too much carb)	_____

SNACKS:

Time: _____ Details: _____

Time: _____ Details: _____

Time: _____ Details: _____

DRINKS:

Details: _____

_____

_____

LIFESTYLE:

What time did you go to sleep? _____   What time did you get up? _____

Sleep quality? ☐ Sound ☐ Restless   Did you have night Sweats? ☐ Yes ☐ No

Did you awake during night (give time & reason)? _____

Did you wake up refreshed today or tired? ☐ Refreshed ☐ Tired

Did you start slow this morning? ☐ Yes ☐ No   If yes, how long did it take to feel alert? _____

Bowel movement(s)?

(number, colour, size & shape)

_____

_____

MOVEMENT :

Details: _____

_____

_____

GENERAL:

How did you feel today? _____

_____

_____

OTHER INFO: _____

DAILY FOOD & LIFESTYLE DIARY

DAILY FOOD DIARY - DATE: _____   Complete everyday for 12 weeks

MEAL 1 – TIME: _____   Please fill out form 1-2 hours after each meal

Most likely too many carbs	Balanced Responses	Most likely too much protein &/or fat	
☐ Headache	☐ Appetite feels satisfied	☐ Lethargic	Approx. of macro Nutrient ratios of meal
☐ Anxiety	☐ Feel emotionally balanced	☐ Mentally Sluggish	% Carbs _____
☐ Jittery/wired	☐ Good mental focus	☐ Heavy Gut	% Protein _____
☐ Difficulty concentrating	☐ Normal level of energy	☐ Feel full yet still hungry	% Fat _____
☐ Hunger is not satisfied	☐ No cravings for sweets	☐ Crave sweets	Foods Eaten: _____
☐ Crave sweet	☐ No cravings for more food	☐ Crave Caffeine	_____
☐ Crave Protein & fat		(if more than hour after meal could	_____
		be a crash from too much carb)	_____

MEAL 2 – TIME: _____

Most likely too many carbs	Balanced Responses	Most likely too much protein &/or fat	
☐ Headache	☐ Appetite feels satisfied	☐ Lethargic	Approx. of macro Nutrient ratios of meal
☐ Anxiety	☐ Feel emotionally balanced	☐ Mentally Sluggish	% Carbs _____
☐ Jittery/wired	☐ Good mental focus	☐ Heavy Gut	% Protein _____
☐ Difficulty concentrating	☐ Normal level of energy	☐ Feel full yet still hungry	% Fat _____
☐ Hunger is not satisfied	☐ No cravings for sweets	☐ Crave sweets	Foods Eaten: _____
☐ Crave sweet	☐ No cravings for more food	☐ Crave Caffeine	_____
☐ Crave Protein & fat		(if more than hour after meal could	_____
		be a crash from too much carb)	_____

MEAL 3 – TIME: _____

Most likely too many carbs	Balanced Responses	Most likely too much protein &/or fat	
☐ Headache	☐ Appetite feels satisfied	☐ Lethargic	Approx. of macro Nutrient ratios of meal
☐ Anxiety	☐ Feel emotionally balanced	☐ Mentally Sluggish	% Carbs _____
☐ Jittery/wired	☐ Good mental focus	☐ Heavy Gut	% Protein _____
☐ Difficulty concentrating	☐ Normal level of energy	☐ Feel full yet still hungry	% Fat _____
☐ Hunger is not satisfied	☐ No cravings for sweets	☐ Crave sweets	Foods Eaten: _____
☐ Crave sweet	☐ No cravings for more food	☐ Crave Caffeine	_____
☐ Crave Protein & fat		(if more than hour after meal could	_____
		be a crash from too much carb)	_____

SNACKS: **DRINKS:**

Time: _____ Details: _____   Details: _____

Time: _____ Details: _____   _____

Time: _____ Details: _____   _____

LIFESTYLE:

What time did you go to sleep?_____   What time did you get up? _____   Bowel movement(s)?

Sleep quality? ☐ Sound ☐ Restless   Did you have night Sweats? ☐ Yes ☐ No   (number, colour, size & shape)

Did you awake during night (give time & reason)? _____

Did you wake up refreshed today or tired? ☐ Refreshed ☐ Tired

Did you start slow this morning? ☐ Yes ☐ No   If yes, how long did it take to feel alert? _____

MOVEMENT :   **GENERAL:**

Details: _____   How did you feel today? _____

_____   _____

OTHER INFO: _____

DAILY FOOD & LIFESTYLE DIARY

DAILY FOOD DIARY - DATE: _____

Complete everyday for 12 weeks

MEAL 1 – TIME: _____

Please fill out form 1-2 hours after each meal

Most likely too many carbs

☐ Headache
☐ Anxiety
☐ Jittery/wired
☐ Difficulty concentrating
☐ Hunger is not satisfied
☐ Crave sweet
☐ Crave Protein & fat

Balanced Responses

☐ Appetite feels satisfied
☐ Feel emotionally balanced
☐ Good mental focus
☐ Normal level of energy
☐ No cravings for sweets
☐ No cravings for more food

Most likely too much protein &/or fat

☐ Lethargic
☐ Mentally Sluggish
☐ Heavy Gut
☐ Feel full yet still hungry
☐ Crave sweets
☐ Crave Caffeine
(if more than hour after meal could
be a crash from too much carb)

Approx. of macro Nutrient ratios of meal
% Carbs _____
% Protein _____
% Fat _____
Foods Eaten: _____
_____
_____
_____
_____

MEAL 2 – TIME: _____

Most likely too many carbs

☐ Headache
☐ Anxiety
☐ Jittery/wired
☐ Difficulty concentrating
☐ Hunger is not satisfied
☐ Crave sweet
☐ Crave Protein & fat

Balanced Responses

☐ Appetite feels satisfied
☐ Feel emotionally balanced
☐ Good mental focus
☐ Normal level of energy
☐ No cravings for sweets
☐ No cravings for more food

Most likely too much protein &/or fat

☐ Lethargic
☐ Mentally Sluggish
☐ Heavy Gut
☐ Feel full yet still hungry
☐ Crave sweets
☐ Crave Caffeine
(if more than hour after meal could
be a crash from too much carb)

Approx. of macro Nutrient ratios of meal
% Carbs _____
% Protein _____
% Fat _____
Foods Eaten: _____
_____
_____
_____
_____

MEAL 3 – TIME: _____

Most likely too many carbs

☐ Headache
☐ Anxiety
☐ Jittery/wired
☐ Difficulty concentrating
☐ Hunger is not satisfied
☐ Crave sweet
☐ Crave Protein & fat

Balanced Responses

☐ Appetite feels satisfied
☐ Feel emotionally balanced
☐ Good mental focus
☐ Normal level of energy
☐ No cravings for sweets
☐ No cravings for more food

Most likely too much protein &/or fat

☐ Lethargic
☐ Mentally Sluggish
☐ Heavy Gut
☐ Feel full yet still hungry
☐ Crave sweets
☐ Crave Caffeine
(if more than hour after meal could
be a crash from too much carb)

Approx. of macro Nutrient ratios of meal
% Carbs _____
% Protein _____
% Fat _____
Foods Eaten: _____
_____
_____
_____
_____

SNACKS:

Time: _____ Details: _____
Time: _____ Details: _____
Time: _____ Details: _____

DRINKS:

Details: _____
_____
_____

LIFESTYLE:

What time did you go to sleep? _____ What time did you get up? _____
Sleep quality? ☐ Sound ☐ Restless   Did you have night Sweats? ☐ Yes ☐ No
Did you awake during night (give time & reason)? _____
Did you wake up refreshed today or tired? ☐ Refreshed ☐ Tired
Did you start slow this morning? ☐ Yes ☐ No   If yes, how long did it take to feel alert? _____

Bowel movement(s)?
(number, colour, size & shape)
_____
_____

MOVEMENT :

Details: _____
_____
_____

GENERAL:

How did you feel today? _____
_____
_____

OTHER INFO: _____

DAILY FOOD & LIFESTYLE DIARY

DAILY FOOD DIARY - DATE: _____

Complete everyday for 12 weeks

MEAL 1 – TIME: _____

Please fill out form 1-2 hours after each meal

Most likely too many carbs

- ☐ Headache
- ☐ Anxiety
- ☐ Jittery/wired
- ☐ Difficulty concentrating
- ☐ Hunger is not satisfied
- ☐ Crave sweet
- ☐ Crave Protein & fat

Balanced Responses

- ☐ Appetite feels satisfied
- ☐ Feel emotionally balanced
- ☐ Good mental focus
- ☐ Normal level of energy
- ☐ No cravings for sweets
- ☐ No cravings for more food

Most likely too much protein &/or fat

- ☐ Lethargic
- ☐ Mentally Sluggish
- ☐ Heavy Gut
- ☐ Feel full yet still hungry
- ☐ Crave sweets
- ☐ Crave Caffeine

(if more than hour after meal could be a crash from too much carb)

Approx. of macro Nutrient ratios of meal
% Carbs _____
% Protein _____
% Fat _____
Foods Eaten: _____
_____
_____
_____
_____
_____

MEAL 2 – TIME: _____

Most likely too many carbs

- ☐ Headache
- ☐ Anxiety
- ☐ Jittery/wired
- ☐ Difficulty concentrating
- ☐ Hunger is not satisfied
- ☐ Crave sweet
- ☐ Crave Protein & fat

Balanced Responses

- ☐ Appetite feels satisfied
- ☐ Feel emotionally balanced
- ☐ Good mental focus
- ☐ Normal level of energy
- ☐ No cravings for sweets
- ☐ No cravings for more food

Most likely too much protein &/or fat

- ☐ Lethargic
- ☐ Mentally Sluggish
- ☐ Heavy Gut
- ☐ Feel full yet still hungry
- ☐ Crave sweets
- ☐ Crave Caffeine

(if more than hour after meal could be a crash from too much carb)

Approx. of macro Nutrient ratios of meal
% Carbs _____
% Protein _____
% Fat _____
Foods Eaten: _____
_____
_____
_____
_____
_____

MEAL 3 – TIME: _____

Most likely too many carbs

- ☐ Headache
- ☐ Anxiety
- ☐ Jittery/wired
- ☐ Difficulty concentrating
- ☐ Hunger is not satisfied
- ☐ Crave sweet
- ☐ Crave Protein & fat

Balanced Responses

- ☐ Appetite feels satisfied
- ☐ Feel emotionally balanced
- ☐ Good mental focus
- ☐ Normal level of energy
- ☐ No cravings for sweets
- ☐ No cravings for more food

Most likely too much protein &/or fat

- ☐ Lethargic
- ☐ Mentally Sluggish
- ☐ Heavy Gut
- ☐ Feel full yet still hungry
- ☐ Crave sweets
- ☐ Crave Caffeine

(if more than hour after meal could be a crash from too much carb)

Approx. of macro Nutrient ratios of meal
% Carbs _____
% Protein _____
% Fat _____
Foods Eaten: _____
_____
_____
_____
_____
_____

SNACKS:

Time: _____ Details: _____
Time: _____ Details: _____
Time: _____ Details: _____

DRINKS:

Details: _____
_____
_____

LIFESTYLE:

What time did you go to sleep?_____ What time did you get up? _____ Bowel movement(s)?
Sleep quality? ☐ Sound ☐ Restless Did you have night Sweats? ☐ Yes ☐ No (number, colour, size & shape)
Did you awake during night (give time & reason)? _____ _____
Did you wake up refreshed today or tired? ☐ Refreshed ☐ Tired _____
Did you start slow this morning? ☐ Yes ☐ No   If yes, how long did it take to feel alert? _____

MOVEMENT :

Details:_____
_____
_____

GENERAL:

How did you feel today? _____
_____
_____

OTHER INFO: _____

DAILY FOOD & LIFESTYLE DIARY

DAILY FOOD DIARY - DATE: _____

Complete everyday for 12 weeks

MEAL 1 – TIME: _____

Please fill out form 1-2 hours after each meal

Most likely too many carbs

☐ Headache
☐ Anxiety
☐ Jittery/wired
☐ Difficulty concentrating
☐ Hunger is not satisfied
☐ Crave sweet
☐ Crave Protein & fat

Balanced Responses

☐ Appetite feels satisfied
☐ Feel emotionally balanced
☐ Good mental focus
☐ Normal level of energy
☐ No cravings for sweets
☐ No cravings for more food

Most likely too much protein &/or fat

☐ Lethargic
☐ Mentally Sluggish
☐ Heavy Gut
☐ Feel full yet still hungry
☐ Crave sweets
☐ Crave Caffeine
(if more than hour after meal could
be a crash from too much carb)

Approx. of macro Nutrient ratios of meal
% Carbs _____
% Protein _____
% Fat _____
Foods Eaten: _____
_____
_____
_____
_____
_____

MEAL 2 – TIME: _____

Most likely too many carbs

☐ Headache
☐ Anxiety
☐ Jittery/wired
☐ Difficulty concentrating
☐ Hunger is not satisfied
☐ Crave sweet
☐ Crave Protein & fat

Balanced Responses

☐ Appetite feels satisfied
☐ Feel emotionally balanced
☐ Good mental focus
☐ Normal level of energy
☐ No cravings for sweets
☐ No cravings for more food

Most likely too much protein &/or fat

☐ Lethargic
☐ Mentally Sluggish
☐ Heavy Gut
☐ Feel full yet still hungry
☐ Crave sweets
☐ Crave Caffeine
(if more than hour after meal could
be a crash from too much carb)

Approx. of macro Nutrient ratios of meal
% Carbs _____
% Protein _____
% Fat _____
Foods Eaten: _____
_____
_____
_____
_____
_____

MEAL 3 – TIME: _____

Most likely too many carbs

☐ Headache
☐ Anxiety
☐ Jittery/wired
☐ Difficulty concentrating
☐ Hunger is not satisfied
☐ Crave sweet
☐ Crave Protein & fat

Balanced Responses

☐ Appetite feels satisfied
☐ Feel emotionally balanced
☐ Good mental focus
☐ Normal level of energy
☐ No cravings for sweets
☐ No cravings for more food

Most likely too much protein &/or fat

☐ Lethargic
☐ Mentally Sluggish
☐ Heavy Gut
☐ Feel full yet still hungry
☐ Crave sweets
☐ Crave Caffeine
(if more than hour after meal could
be a crash from too much carb)

Approx. of macro Nutrient ratios of meal
% Carbs _____
% Protein _____
% Fat _____
Foods Eaten: _____
_____
_____
_____
_____
_____

SNACKS:

Time: _____ Details: _____
Time: _____ Details: _____
Time: _____ Details: _____

DRINKS:

Details: _____
_____
_____

LIFESTYLE:

What time did you go to sleep? _____ What time did you get up? _____
Sleep quality? ☐ Sound ☐ Restless   Did you have night Sweats? ☐ Yes ☐ No
Did you awake during night (give time & reason)? _____
Did you wake up refreshed today or tired? ☐ Refreshed ☐ Tired
Did you start slow this morning? ☐ Yes ☐ No   If yes, how long did it take to feel alert? _____

Bowel movement(s)?
(number, colour, size & shape)
_____
_____

MOVEMENT :

Details: _____
_____
_____

GENERAL:

How did you feel today? _____
_____
_____

OTHER INFO: _____

DAILY FOOD & LIFESTYLE DIARY

DAILY FOOD DIARY - DATE: _____

Complete everyday for 12 weeks

MEAL 1 – TIME: _____

Please fill out form 1-2 hours after each meal

Most likely too many carbs	Balanced Responses	Most likely too much protein &/or fat	
☐ Headache	☐ Appetite feels satisfied	☐ Lethargic	Approx. of macro Nutrient ratios of meal
☐ Anxiety	☐ Feel emotionally balanced	☐ Mentally Sluggish	% Carbs _____
☐ Jittery/wired	☐ Good mental focus	☐ Heavy Gut	% Protein _____
☐ Difficulty concentrating	☐ Normal level of energy	☐ Feel full yet still hungry	% Fat _____
☐ Hunger is not satisfied	☐ No cravings for sweets	☐ Crave sweets	Foods Eaten: _____
☐ Crave sweet	☐ No cravings for more food	☐ Crave Caffeine	_____
☐ Crave Protein & fat		(if more than hour after meal could be a crash from too much carb)	_____

MEAL 2 – TIME: _____

Most likely too many carbs	Balanced Responses	Most likely too much protein &/or fat	
☐ Headache	☐ Appetite feels satisfied	☐ Lethargic	Approx. of macro Nutrient ratios of meal
☐ Anxiety	☐ Feel emotionally balanced	☐ Mentally Sluggish	% Carbs _____
☐ Jittery/wired	☐ Good mental focus	☐ Heavy Gut	% Protein _____
☐ Difficulty concentrating	☐ Normal level of energy	☐ Feel full yet still hungry	% Fat _____
☐ Hunger is not satisfied	☐ No cravings for sweets	☐ Crave sweets	Foods Eaten: _____
☐ Crave sweet	☐ No cravings for more food	☐ Crave Caffeine	_____
☐ Crave Protein & fat		(if more than hour after meal could be a crash from too much carb)	_____

MEAL 3 – TIME: _____

Most likely too many carbs	Balanced Responses	Most likely too much protein &/or fat	
☐ Headache	☐ Appetite feels satisfied	☐ Lethargic	Approx. of macro Nutrient ratios of meal
☐ Anxiety	☐ Feel emotionally balanced	☐ Mentally Sluggish	% Carbs _____
☐ Jittery/wired	☐ Good mental focus	☐ Heavy Gut	% Protein _____
☐ Difficulty concentrating	☐ Normal level of energy	☐ Feel full yet still hungry	% Fat _____
☐ Hunger is not satisfied	☐ No cravings for sweets	☐ Crave sweets	Foods Eaten: _____
☐ Crave sweet	☐ No cravings for more food	☐ Crave Caffeine	_____
☐ Crave Protein & fat		(if more than hour after meal could be a crash from too much carb)	_____

SNACKS:

Time: _____ Details: _____
Time: _____ Details: _____
Time: _____ Details: _____

DRINKS:

Details: _____
_____
_____

LIFESTYLE:

What time did you go to sleep? _____ What time did you get up? _____

Sleep quality? ☐ Sound ☐ Restless   Did you have night Sweats? ☐ Yes ☐ No

Bowel movement(s)?
(number, colour, size & shape)
_____
_____

Did you awake during night (give time & reason)? _____

Did you wake up refreshed today or tired? ☐ Refreshed ☐ Tired

Did you start slow this morning? ☐ Yes ☐ No   If yes, how long did it take to feel alert? _____

MOVEMENT :

Details: _____
_____
_____

GENERAL:

How did you feel today? _____
_____
_____

OTHER INFO: _____

DAILY FOOD & LIFESTYLE DIARY

DAILY FOOD DIARY - DATE: _____

Complete everyday for 12 weeks

MEAL 1 – TIME: _____

Please fill out form 1-2 hours after each meal

Most likely too many carbs	Balanced Responses	Most likely too much protein &/or fat	
☐ Headache	☐ Appetite feels satisfied	☐ Lethargic	Approx. of macro Nutrient ratios of meal
☐ Anxiety	☐ Feel emotionally balanced	☐ Mentally Sluggish	% Carbs _____
☐ Jittery/wired	☐ Good mental focus	☐ Heavy Gut	% Protein _____
☐ Difficulty concentrating	☐ Normal level of energy	☐ Feel full yet still hungry	% Fat _____
☐ Hunger is not satisfied	☐ No cravings for sweets	☐ Crave sweets	Foods Eaten: _____
☐ Crave sweet	☐ No cravings for more food	☐ Crave Caffeine	_____
☐ Crave Protein & fat		(if more than hour after meal could	_____
		be a crash from too much carb)	_____
			_____
			_____

MEAL 2 – TIME: _____

Most likely too many carbs	Balanced Responses	Most likely too much protein &/or fat	
☐ Headache	☐ Appetite feels satisfied	☐ Lethargic	Approx. of macro Nutrient ratios of meal
☐ Anxiety	☐ Feel emotionally balanced	☐ Mentally Sluggish	% Carbs _____
☐ Jittery/wired	☐ Good mental focus	☐ Heavy Gut	% Protein _____
☐ Difficulty concentrating	☐ Normal level of energy	☐ Feel full yet still hungry	% Fat _____
☐ Hunger is not satisfied	☐ No cravings for sweets	☐ Crave sweets	Foods Eaten: _____
☐ Crave sweet	☐ No cravings for more food	☐ Crave Caffeine	_____
☐ Crave Protein & fat		(if more than hour after meal could	_____
		be a crash from too much carb)	_____
			_____
			_____

MEAL 3 – TIME: _____

Most likely too many carbs	Balanced Responses	Most likely too much protein &/or fat	
☐ Headache	☐ Appetite feels satisfied	☐ Lethargic	Approx. of macro Nutrient ratios of meal
☐ Anxiety	☐ Feel emotionally balanced	☐ Mentally Sluggish	% Carbs _____
☐ Jittery/wired	☐ Good mental focus	☐ Heavy Gut	% Protein _____
☐ Difficulty concentrating	☐ Normal level of energy	☐ Feel full yet still hungry	% Fat _____
☐ Hunger is not satisfied	☐ No cravings for sweets	☐ Crave sweets	Foods Eaten: _____
☐ Crave sweet	☐ No cravings for more food	☐ Crave Caffeine	_____
☐ Crave Protein & fat		(if more than hour after meal could	_____
		be a crash from too much carb)	_____
			_____
			_____

SNACKS:

Time: _____ Details: _____
Time: _____ Details: _____
Time: _____ Details: _____

DRINKS:

Details: _____
_____
_____

LIFESTYLE:

What time did you go to sleep? _____ What time did you get up? _____ Bowel movement(s)?
Sleep quality? ☐ Sound ☐ Restless   Did you have night Sweats? ☐ Yes ☐ No   (number, colour, size & shape)
Did you awake during night (give time & reason)? _____ _____
Did you wake up refreshed today or tired? ☐ Refreshed ☐ Tired _____
Did you start slow this morning? ☐ Yes ☐ No   If yes, how long did it take to feel alert? _____

MOVEMENT :

Details: _____
_____

GENERAL:

How did you feel today? _____
_____

OTHER INFO: _____

DAILY FOOD & LIFESTYLE DIARY

DAILY FOOD DIARY - DATE: _____

Complete everyday for 12 weeks

MEAL 1 – TIME: _____

Please fill out form 1-2 hours after each meal

Most likely too many carbs	Balanced Responses	Most likely too much protein &/or fat	
☐ Headache	☐ Appetite feels satisfied	☐ Lethargic	Approx. of macro Nutrient ratios of meal
☐ Anxiety	☐ Feel emotionally balanced	☐ Mentally Sluggish	% Carbs _____
☐ Jittery/wired	☐ Good mental focus	☐ Heavy Gut	% Protein _____
☐ Difficulty concentrating	☐ Normal level of energy	☐ Feel full yet still hungry	% Fat _____
☐ Hunger is not satisfied	☐ No cravings for sweets	☐ Crave sweets	Foods Eaten: _____
☐ Crave sweet	☐ No cravings for more food	☐ Crave Caffeine	_____
☐ Crave Protein & fat		(if more than hour after meal could	_____
		be a crash from too much carb)	_____
			_____
			_____

MEAL 2 – TIME: _____

Most likely too many carbs	Balanced Responses	Most likely too much protein &/or fat	
☐ Headache	☐ Appetite feels satisfied	☐ Lethargic	Approx. of macro Nutrient ratios of meal
☐ Anxiety	☐ Feel emotionally balanced	☐ Mentally Sluggish	% Carbs _____
☐ Jittery/wired	☐ Good mental focus	☐ Heavy Gut	% Protein _____
☐ Difficulty concentrating	☐ Normal level of energy	☐ Feel full yet still hungry	% Fat _____
☐ Hunger is not satisfied	☐ No cravings for sweets	☐ Crave sweets	Foods Eaten: _____
☐ Crave sweet	☐ No cravings for more food	☐ Crave Caffeine	_____
☐ Crave Protein & fat		(if more than hour after meal could	_____
		be a crash from too much carb)	_____
			_____
			_____

MEAL 3 – TIME: _____

Most likely too many carbs	Balanced Responses	Most likely too much protein &/or fat	
☐ Headache	☐ Appetite feels satisfied	☐ Lethargic	Approx. of macro Nutrient ratios of meal
☐ Anxiety	☐ Feel emotionally balanced	☐ Mentally Sluggish	% Carbs _____
☐ Jittery/wired	☐ Good mental focus	☐ Heavy Gut	% Protein _____
☐ Difficulty concentrating	☐ Normal level of energy	☐ Feel full yet still hungry	% Fat _____
☐ Hunger is not satisfied	☐ No cravings for sweets	☐ Crave sweets	Foods Eaten: _____
☐ Crave sweet	☐ No cravings for more food	☐ Crave Caffeine	_____
☐ Crave Protein & fat		(if more than hour after meal could	_____
		be a crash from too much carb)	_____
			_____
			_____

SNACKS:

Time: _____ Details: _____
Time: _____ Details: _____
Time: _____ Details: _____

DRINKS:

Details: _____
_____
_____

LIFESTYLE:

What time did you go to sleep?_____ What time did you get up? _____ Bowel movement(s)?
Sleep quality? ☐ Sound ☐ Restless   Did you have night Sweats? ☐ Yes ☐ No   (number, colour, size & shape)
Did you awake during night (give time & reason)? _____
Did you wake up refreshed today or tired? ☐ Refreshed ☐ Tired
Did you start slow this morning? ☐ Yes ☐ No   If yes, how long did it take to feel alert? _____

MOVEMENT :

Details: _____
_____
_____

GENERAL:

How did you feel today? _____
_____

OTHER INFO: _____

DAILY FOOD & LIFESTYLE DIARY

DAILY FOOD DIARY - DATE: _____

Complete everyday for 12 weeks

MEAL 1 – TIME: _____

Please fill out form 1-2 hours after each meal

Most likely too many carbs	Balanced Responses	Most likely too much protein &/or fat	Approx. of macro Nutrient ratios of meal
☐ Headache	☐ Appetite feels satisfied	☐ Lethargic	% Carbs _____
☐ Anxiety	☐ Feel emotionally balanced	☐ Mentally Sluggish	% Protein _____
☐ Jittery/wired	☐ Good mental focus	☐ Heavy Gut	% Fat _____
☐ Difficulty concentrating	☐ Normal level of energy	☐ Feel full yet still hungry	Foods Eaten: _____
☐ Hunger is not satisfied	☐ No cravings for sweets	☐ Crave sweets	_____
☐ Crave sweet	☐ No cravings for more food	☐ Crave Caffeine	_____
☐ Crave Protein & fat		(if more than hour after meal could be a crash from too much carb)	_____

MEAL 2 – TIME: _____

Most likely too many carbs	Balanced Responses	Most likely too much protein &/or fat	Approx. of macro Nutrient ratios of meal
☐ Headache	☐ Appetite feels satisfied	☐ Lethargic	% Carbs _____
☐ Anxiety	☐ Feel emotionally balanced	☐ Mentally Sluggish	% Protein _____
☐ Jittery/wired	☐ Good mental focus	☐ Heavy Gut	% Fat _____
☐ Difficulty concentrating	☐ Normal level of energy	☐ Feel full yet still hungry	Foods Eaten: _____
☐ Hunger is not satisfied	☐ No cravings for sweets	☐ Crave sweets	_____
☐ Crave sweet	☐ No cravings for more food	☐ Crave Caffeine	_____
☐ Crave Protein & fat		(if more than hour after meal could be a crash from too much carb)	_____

MEAL 3 – TIME: _____

Most likely too many carbs	Balanced Responses	Most likely too much protein &/or fat	Approx. of macro Nutrient ratios of meal
☐ Headache	☐ Appetite feels satisfied	☐ Lethargic	% Carbs _____
☐ Anxiety	☐ Feel emotionally balanced	☐ Mentally Sluggish	% Protein _____
☐ Jittery/wired	☐ Good mental focus	☐ Heavy Gut	% Fat _____
☐ Difficulty concentrating	☐ Normal level of energy	☐ Feel full yet still hungry	Foods Eaten: _____
☐ Hunger is not satisfied	☐ No cravings for sweets	☐ Crave sweets	_____
☐ Crave sweet	☐ No cravings for more food	☐ Crave Caffeine	_____
☐ Crave Protein & fat		(if more than hour after meal could be a crash from too much carb)	_____

SNACKS:

Time: _____ Details: _____
Time: _____ Details: _____
Time: _____ Details: _____

DRINKS:

Details: _____
_____
_____

LIFESTYLE:

What time did you go to sleep? _____ What time did you get up? _____
Sleep quality? ☐ Sound ☐ Restless   Did you have night Sweats? ☐ Yes ☐ No
Did you awake during night (give time & reason)? _____
Did you wake up refreshed today or tired? ☐ Refreshed ☐ Tired
Did you start slow this morning? ☐ Yes ☐ No   If yes, how long did it take to feel alert? _____

Bowel movement(s)?
(number, colour, size & shape)
_____
_____

MOVEMENT :

Details: _____
_____
_____

GENERAL:

How did you feel today? _____
_____
_____

OTHER INFO: _____

DAILY FOOD & LIFESTYLE DIARY

DAILY FOOD DIARY - DATE: _____

Complete everyday for 12 weeks

MEAL 1 – TIME: _____

Please fill out form 1-2 hours after each meal

Most likely too many carbs	Balanced Responses	Most likely too much protein &/or fat	
☐ Headache	☐ Appetite feels satisfied	☐ Lethargic	Approx. of macro Nutrient ratios of meal
☐ Anxiety	☐ Feel emotionally balanced	☐ Mentally Sluggish	% Carbs _____
☐ Jittery/wired	☐ Good mental focus	☐ Heavy Gut	% Protein _____
☐ Difficulty concentrating	☐ Normal level of energy	☐ Feel full yet still hungry	% Fat _____
☐ Hunger is not satisfied	☐ No cravings for sweets	☐ Crave sweets	Foods Eaten: _____
☐ Crave sweet	☐ No cravings for more food	☐ Crave Caffeine	_____
☐ Crave Protein & fat		(if more than hour after meal could be a crash from too much carb)	_____

MEAL 2 – TIME: _____

Most likely too many carbs	Balanced Responses	Most likely too much protein &/or fat	
☐ Headache	☐ Appetite feels satisfied	☐ Lethargic	Approx. of macro Nutrient ratios of meal
☐ Anxiety	☐ Feel emotionally balanced	☐ Mentally Sluggish	% Carbs _____
☐ Jittery/wired	☐ Good mental focus	☐ Heavy Gut	% Protein _____
☐ Difficulty concentrating	☐ Normal level of energy	☐ Feel full yet still hungry	% Fat _____
☐ Hunger is not satisfied	☐ No cravings for sweets	☐ Crave sweets	Foods Eaten: _____
☐ Crave sweet	☐ No cravings for more food	☐ Crave Caffeine	_____
☐ Crave Protein & fat		(if more than hour after meal could be a crash from too much carb)	_____

MEAL 3 – TIME: _____

Most likely too many carbs	Balanced Responses	Most likely too much protein &/or fat	
☐ Headache	☐ Appetite feels satisfied	☐ Lethargic	Approx. of macro Nutrient ratios of meal
☐ Anxiety	☐ Feel emotionally balanced	☐ Mentally Sluggish	% Carbs _____
☐ Jittery/wired	☐ Good mental focus	☐ Heavy Gut	% Protein _____
☐ Difficulty concentrating	☐ Normal level of energy	☐ Feel full yet still hungry	% Fat _____
☐ Hunger is not satisfied	☐ No cravings for sweets	☐ Crave sweets	Foods Eaten: _____
☐ Crave sweet	☐ No cravings for more food	☐ Crave Caffeine	_____
☐ Crave Protein & fat		(if more than hour after meal could be a crash from too much carb)	_____

SNACKS:

Time: _____ Details: _____
Time: _____ Details: _____
Time: _____ Details: _____

DRINKS:

Details: _____
_____
_____

LIFESTYLE:

What time did you go to sleep?_____ What time did you get up? _____

Sleep quality? ☐ Sound ☐ Restless   Did you have night Sweats? ☐ Yes ☐ No

Did you awake during night (give time & reason)? _____

Did you wake up refreshed today or tired? ☐ Refreshed ☐ Tired

Did you start slow this morning? ☐ Yes ☐ No   If yes, how long did it take to feel alert? _____

Bowel movement(s)?
(number, colour, size & shape)

_____
_____

MOVEMENT :

Details: _____
_____
_____

GENERAL:

How did you feel today? _____
_____
_____

OTHER INFO: _____

DAILY FOOD & LIFESTYLE DIARY

DAILY FOOD DIARY - DATE: _____

Complete everyday for 12 weeks

MEAL 1 – TIME: _____

Please fill out form 1-2 hours after each meal

Most likely too many carbs

- ☐ Headache
- ☐ Anxiety
- ☐ Jittery/wired
- ☐ Difficulty concentrating
- ☐ Hunger is not satisfied
- ☐ Crave sweet
- ☐ Crave Protein & fat

Balanced Responses

- ☐ Appetite feels satisfied
- ☐ Feel emotionally balanced
- ☐ Good mental focus
- ☐ Normal level of energy
- ☐ No cravings for sweets
- ☐ No cravings for more food

Most likely too much protein &/or fat

- ☐ Lethargic
- ☐ Mentally Sluggish
- ☐ Heavy Gut
- ☐ Feel full yet still hungry
- ☐ Crave sweets
- ☐ Crave Caffeine

(if more than hour after meal could be a crash from too much carb)

Approx. of macro Nutrient ratios of meal
% Carbs _____
% Protein _____
% Fat _____
Foods Eaten: _____
_____
_____
_____
_____
_____

MEAL 2 – TIME: _____

Most likely too many carbs

- ☐ Headache
- ☐ Anxiety
- ☐ Jittery/wired
- ☐ Difficulty concentrating
- ☐ Hunger is not satisfied
- ☐ Crave sweet
- ☐ Crave Protein & fat

Balanced Responses

- ☐ Appetite feels satisfied
- ☐ Feel emotionally balanced
- ☐ Good mental focus
- ☐ Normal level of energy
- ☐ No cravings for sweets
- ☐ No cravings for more food

Most likely too much protein &/or fat

- ☐ Lethargic
- ☐ Mentally Sluggish
- ☐ Heavy Gut
- ☐ Feel full yet still hungry
- ☐ Crave sweets
- ☐ Crave Caffeine

(if more than hour after meal could be a crash from too much carb)

Approx. of macro Nutrient ratios of meal
% Carbs _____
% Protein _____
% Fat _____
Foods Eaten: _____
_____
_____
_____
_____
_____

MEAL 3 – TIME: _____

Most likely too many carbs

- ☐ Headache
- ☐ Anxiety
- ☐ Jittery/wired
- ☐ Difficulty concentrating
- ☐ Hunger is not satisfied
- ☐ Crave sweet
- ☐ Crave Protein & fat

Balanced Responses

- ☐ Appetite feels satisfied
- ☐ Feel emotionally balanced
- ☐ Good mental focus
- ☐ Normal level of energy
- ☐ No cravings for sweets
- ☐ No cravings for more food

Most likely too much protein &/or fat

- ☐ Lethargic
- ☐ Mentally Sluggish
- ☐ Heavy Gut
- ☐ Feel full yet still hungry
- ☐ Crave sweets
- ☐ Crave Caffeine

(if more than hour after meal could be a crash from too much carb)

Approx. of macro Nutrient ratios of meal
% Carbs _____
% Protein _____
% Fat _____
Foods Eaten: _____
_____
_____
_____
_____
_____

SNACKS:

Time: _____ Details: _____
Time: _____ Details: _____
Time: _____ Details: _____

DRINKS:

Details: _____
_____
_____

LIFESTYLE:

What time did you go to sleep? _____   What time did you get up? _____
Sleep quality? ☐ Sound ☐ Restless   Did you have night Sweats? ☐ Yes ☐ No
Did you awake during night (give time & reason)? _____
Did you wake up refreshed today or tired? ☐ Refreshed ☐ Tired
Did you start slow this morning? ☐ Yes ☐ No   If yes, how long did it take to feel alert? _____

Bowel movement(s)?
(number, colour, size & shape)
_____
_____

MOVEMENT :

Details: _____
_____
_____

GENERAL:

How did you feel today? _____
_____
_____

OTHER INFO: _____

175

DAILY FOOD & LIFESTYLE DIARY

DAILY FOOD DIARY - DATE: _____

Complete everyday for 12 weeks

MEAL 1 – TIME: _____

Please fill out form 1-2 hours after each meal

Most likely too many carbs	Balanced Responses	Most likely too much protein &/or fat	
☐ Headache	☐ Appetite feels satisfied	☐ Lethargic	Approx. of macro Nutrient ratios of meal
☐ Anxiety	☐ Feel emotionally balanced	☐ Mentally Sluggish	% Carbs _____
☐ Jittery/wired	☐ Good mental focus	☐ Heavy Gut	% Protein _____
☐ Difficulty concentrating	☐ Normal level of energy	☐ Feel full yet still hungry	% Fat _____
☐ Hunger is not satisfied	☐ No cravings for sweets	☐ Crave sweets	Foods Eaten: _____
☐ Crave sweet	☐ No cravings for more food	☐ Crave Caffeine	_____
☐ Crave Protein & fat		(if more than hour after meal could	_____
		be a crash from too much carb)	_____

MEAL 2 – TIME: _____

Most likely too many carbs	Balanced Responses	Most likely too much protein &/or fat	
☐ Headache	☐ Appetite feels satisfied	☐ Lethargic	Approx. of macro Nutrient ratios of meal
☐ Anxiety	☐ Feel emotionally balanced	☐ Mentally Sluggish	% Carbs _____
☐ Jittery/wired	☐ Good mental focus	☐ Heavy Gut	% Protein _____
☐ Difficulty concentrating	☐ Normal level of energy	☐ Feel full yet still hungry	% Fat _____
☐ Hunger is not satisfied	☐ No cravings for sweets	☐ Crave sweets	Foods Eaten: _____
☐ Crave sweet	☐ No cravings for more food	☐ Crave Caffeine	_____
☐ Crave Protein & fat		(if more than hour after meal could	_____
		be a crash from too much carb)	_____

MEAL 3 – TIME: _____

Most likely too many carbs	Balanced Responses	Most likely too much protein &/or fat	
☐ Headache	☐ Appetite feels satisfied	☐ Lethargic	Approx. of macro Nutrient ratios of meal
☐ Anxiety	☐ Feel emotionally balanced	☐ Mentally Sluggish	% Carbs _____
☐ Jittery/wired	☐ Good mental focus	☐ Heavy Gut	% Protein _____
☐ Difficulty concentrating	☐ Normal level of energy	☐ Feel full yet still hungry	% Fat _____
☐ Hunger is not satisfied	☐ No cravings for sweets	☐ Crave sweets	Foods Eaten: _____
☐ Crave sweet	☐ No cravings for more food	☐ Crave Caffeine	_____
☐ Crave Protein & fat		(if more than hour after meal could	_____
		be a crash from too much carb)	_____

SNACKS:

Time: _____ Details: _____

Time: _____ Details: _____

Time: _____ Details: _____

DRINKS:

Details: _____

_____

LIFESTYLE:

What time did you go to sleep? _____ What time did you get up? _____

Sleep quality? ☐ Sound ☐ Restless   Did you have night Sweats? ☐ Yes ☐ No

Did you awake during night (give time & reason)? _____

Did you wake up refreshed today or tired? ☐ Refreshed ☐ Tired

Did you start slow this morning? ☐ Yes ☐ No   If yes, how long did it take to feel alert? _____

Bowel movement(s)?

(number, colour, size & shape)

_____

MOVEMENT :

Details: _____

_____

GENERAL:

How did you feel today? _____

_____

OTHER INFO: _____

DAILY FOOD & LIFESTYLE DIARY

DAILY FOOD DIARY - DATE: _____

Complete everyday for 12 weeks

MEAL 1 – TIME: _____

Please fill out form 1-2 hours after each meal

Most likely too many carbs	Balanced Responses	Most likely too much protein &/or fat	
☐ Headache	☐ Appetite feels satisfied	☐ Lethargic	Approx. of macro Nutrient ratios of meal
☐ Anxiety	☐ Feel emotionally balanced	☐ Mentally Sluggish	% Carbs _____
☐ Jittery/wired	☐ Good mental focus	☐ Heavy Gut	% Protein _____
☐ Difficulty concentrating	☐ Normal level of energy	☐ Feel full yet still hungry	% Fat _____
☐ Hunger is not satisfied	☐ No cravings for sweets	☐ Crave sweets	Foods Eaten: _____
☐ Crave sweet	☐ No cravings for more food	☐ Crave Caffeine	_____
☐ Crave Protein & fat		(if more than hour after meal could	_____
		be a crash from too much carb)	_____
			_____

MEAL 2 – TIME: _____

Most likely too many carbs	Balanced Responses	Most likely too much protein &/or fat	
☐ Headache	☐ Appetite feels satisfied	☐ Lethargic	Approx. of macro Nutrient ratios of meal
☐ Anxiety	☐ Feel emotionally balanced	☐ Mentally Sluggish	% Carbs _____
☐ Jittery/wired	☐ Good mental focus	☐ Heavy Gut	% Protein _____
☐ Difficulty concentrating	☐ Normal level of energy	☐ Feel full yet still hungry	% Fat _____
☐ Hunger is not satisfied	☐ No cravings for sweets	☐ Crave sweets	Foods Eaten: _____
☐ Crave sweet	☐ No cravings for more food	☐ Crave Caffeine	_____
☐ Crave Protein & fat		(if more than hour after meal could	_____
		be a crash from too much carb)	_____
			_____

MEAL 3 – TIME: _____

Most likely too many carbs	Balanced Responses	Most likely too much protein &/or fat	
☐ Headache	☐ Appetite feels satisfied	☐ Lethargic	Approx. of macro Nutrient ratios of meal
☐ Anxiety	☐ Feel emotionally balanced	☐ Mentally Sluggish	% Carbs _____
☐ Jittery/wired	☐ Good mental focus	☐ Heavy Gut	% Protein _____
☐ Difficulty concentrating	☐ Normal level of energy	☐ Feel full yet still hungry	% Fat _____
☐ Hunger is not satisfied	☐ No cravings for sweets	☐ Crave sweets	Foods Eaten: _____
☐ Crave sweet	☐ No cravings for more food	☐ Crave Caffeine	_____
☐ Crave Protein & fat		(if more than hour after meal could	_____
		be a crash from too much carb)	_____
			_____

SNACKS:

Time: _____ Details: _____
Time: _____ Details: _____
Time: _____ Details: _____

DRINKS:

Details: _____
_____
_____

LIFESTYLE:

What time did you go to sleep? _____ What time did you get up? _____

Sleep quality? ☐ Sound ☐ Restless   Did you have night Sweats? ☐ Yes ☐ No

Did you awake during night (give time & reason)? _____

Did you wake up refreshed today or tired? ☐ Refreshed ☐ Tired

Did you start slow this morning? ☐ Yes ☐ No   If yes, how long did it take to feel alert? _____

Bowel movement(s)?
(number, colour, size & shape)
_____
_____

MOVEMENT :

Details: _____
_____
_____

GENERAL:

How did you feel today? _____
_____
_____

OTHER INFO: _____

DAILY FOOD & LIFESTYLE DIARY

DAILY FOOD DIARY - DATE: _____   Complete everyday for 12 weeks

MEAL 1 – TIME: _____   Please fill out form 1-2 hours after each meal

Most likely too many carbs
- ☐ Headache
- ☐ Anxiety
- ☐ Jittery/wired
- ☐ Difficulty concentrating
- ☐ Hunger is not satisfied
- ☐ Crave sweet
- ☐ Crave Protein & fat

Balanced Responses
- ☐ Appetite feels satisfied
- ☐ Feel emotionally balanced
- ☐ Good mental focus
- ☐ Normal level of energy
- ☐ No cravings for sweets
- ☐ No cravings for more food

Most likely too much protein &/or fat
- ☐ Lethargic
- ☐ Mentally Sluggish
- ☐ Heavy Gut
- ☐ Feel full yet still hungry
- ☐ Crave sweets
- ☐ Crave Caffeine
(if more than hour after meal could be a crash from too much carb)

Approx. of macro Nutrient ratios of meal
% Carbs _____
% Protein _____
% Fat _____
Foods Eaten: _____
_____
_____
_____
_____

MEAL 2 – TIME: _____

Most likely too many carbs
- ☐ Headache
- ☐ Anxiety
- ☐ Jittery/wired
- ☐ Difficulty concentrating
- ☐ Hunger is not satisfied
- ☐ Crave sweet
- ☐ Crave Protein & fat

Balanced Responses
- ☐ Appetite feels satisfied
- ☐ Feel emotionally balanced
- ☐ Good mental focus
- ☐ Normal level of energy
- ☐ No cravings for sweets
- ☐ No cravings for more food

Most likely too much protein &/or fat
- ☐ Lethargic
- ☐ Mentally Sluggish
- ☐ Heavy Gut
- ☐ Feel full yet still hungry
- ☐ Crave sweets
- ☐ Crave Caffeine
(if more than hour after meal could be a crash from too much carb)

Approx. of macro Nutrient ratios of meal
% Carbs _____
% Protein _____
% Fat _____
Foods Eaten: _____
_____
_____
_____
_____

MEAL 3 – TIME: _____

Most likely too many carbs
- ☐ Headache
- ☐ Anxiety
- ☐ Jittery/wired
- ☐ Difficulty concentrating
- ☐ Hunger is not satisfied
- ☐ Crave sweet
- ☐ Crave Protein & fat

Balanced Responses
- ☐ Appetite feels satisfied
- ☐ Feel emotionally balanced
- ☐ Good mental focus
- ☐ Normal level of energy
- ☐ No cravings for sweets
- ☐ No cravings for more food

Most likely too much protein &/or fat
- ☐ Lethargic
- ☐ Mentally Sluggish
- ☐ Heavy Gut
- ☐ Feel full yet still hungry
- ☐ Crave sweets
- ☐ Crave Caffeine
(if more than hour after meal could be a crash from too much carb)

Approx. of macro Nutrient ratios of meal
% Carbs _____
% Protein _____
% Fat _____
Foods Eaten: _____
_____
_____
_____
_____

SNACKS:
Time: _____ Details: _____
Time: _____ Details: _____
Time: _____ Details: _____

DRINKS:
Details: _____
_____
_____

LIFESTYLE:
What time did you go to sleep?_____ What time did you get up? _____   Bowel movement(s)?
Sleep quality? ☐ Sound ☐ Restless   Did you have night Sweats? ☐ Yes ☐ No   (number, colour, size & shape)
Did you awake during night (give time & reason)? _____   _____
Did you wake up refreshed today or tired? ☐ Refreshed ☐ Tired   _____
Did you start slow this morning? ☐ Yes ☐ No   If yes, how long did it take to feel alert? _____

MOVEMENT :
Details: _____
_____
_____

GENERAL:
How did you feel today? _____
_____

OTHER INFO: _____

DAILY FOOD & LIFESTYLE DIARY

DAILY FOOD DIARY - DATE: _____   Complete everyday for 12 weeks

MEAL 1 – TIME: _____   Please fill out form 1-2 hours after each meal

Most likely too many carbs	Balanced Responses	Most likely too much protein &/or fat	
☐ Headache	☐ Appetite feels satisfied	☐ Lethargic	Approx. of macro Nutrient ratios of meal
☐ Anxiety	☐ Feel emotionally balanced	☐ Mentally Sluggish	% Carbs _____
☐ Jittery/wired	☐ Good mental focus	☐ Heavy Gut	% Protein _____
☐ Difficulty concentrating	☐ Normal level of energy	☐ Feel full yet still hungry	% Fat _____
☐ Hunger is not satisfied	☐ No cravings for sweets	☐ Crave sweets	Foods Eaten: _____
☐ Crave sweet	☐ No cravings for more food	☐ Crave Caffeine	_____
☐ Crave Protein & fat		(if more than hour after meal could	_____
		be a crash from too much carb)	_____

MEAL 2 – TIME: _____

Most likely too many carbs	Balanced Responses	Most likely too much protein &/or fat	
☐ Headache	☐ Appetite feels satisfied	☐ Lethargic	Approx. of macro Nutrient ratios of meal
☐ Anxiety	☐ Feel emotionally balanced	☐ Mentally Sluggish	% Carbs _____
☐ Jittery/wired	☐ Good mental focus	☐ Heavy Gut	% Protein _____
☐ Difficulty concentrating	☐ Normal level of energy	☐ Feel full yet still hungry	% Fat _____
☐ Hunger is not satisfied	☐ No cravings for sweets	☐ Crave sweets	Foods Eaten: _____
☐ Crave sweet	☐ No cravings for more food	☐ Crave Caffeine	_____
☐ Crave Protein & fat		(if more than hour after meal could	_____
		be a crash from too much carb)	_____

MEAL 3 – TIME: _____

Most likely too many carbs	Balanced Responses	Most likely too much protein &/or fat	
☐ Headache	☐ Appetite feels satisfied	☐ Lethargic	Approx. of macro Nutrient ratios of meal
☐ Anxiety	☐ Feel emotionally balanced	☐ Mentally Sluggish	% Carbs _____
☐ Jittery/wired	☐ Good mental focus	☐ Heavy Gut	% Protein _____
☐ Difficulty concentrating	☐ Normal level of energy	☐ Feel full yet still hungry	% Fat _____
☐ Hunger is not satisfied	☐ No cravings for sweets	☐ Crave sweets	Foods Eaten: _____
☐ Crave sweet	☐ No cravings for more food	☐ Crave Caffeine	_____
☐ Crave Protein & fat		(if more than hour after meal could	_____
		be a crash from too much carb)	_____

SNACKS:

Time: _____ Details: _____

Time: _____ Details: _____

Time: _____ Details: _____

DRINKS:

Details: _____

_____

_____

LIFESTYLE:

What time did you go to sleep? _____   What time did you get up? _____   Bowel movement(s)?

Sleep quality? ☐ Sound ☐ Restless   Did you have night Sweats? ☐ Yes ☐ No   (number, colour, size & shape)

Did you awake during night (give time & reason)? _____

Did you wake up refreshed today or tired? ☐ Refreshed ☐ Tired

Did you start slow this morning? ☐ Yes ☐ No   If yes, how long did it take to feel alert? _____

MOVEMENT :

Details: _____

_____

_____

GENERAL:

How did you feel today? _____

_____

OTHER INFO: _____

DAILY FOOD & LIFESTYLE DIARY

DAILY FOOD DIARY - DATE: _____

Complete everyday for 12 weeks

MEAL 1 – TIME: _____

Please fill out form 1-2 hours after each meal

Most likely too many carbs	Balanced Responses
☐ Headache	☐ Appetite feels satisfied
☐ Anxiety	☐ Feel emotionally balanced
☐ Jittery/wired	☐ Good mental focus
☐ Difficulty concentrating	☐ Normal level of energy
☐ Hunger is not satisfied	☐ No cravings for sweets
☐ Crave sweet	☐ No cravings for more food
☐ Crave Protein & fat	

Most likely too much protein &/or fat

☐ Lethargic
☐ Mentally Sluggish
☐ Heavy Gut
☐ Feel full yet still hungry
☐ Crave sweets
☐ Crave Caffeine
(if more than hour after meal could be a crash from too much carb)

Approx. of macro Nutrient ratios of meal
% Carbs _____
% Protein _____
% Fat _____
Foods Eaten: _____
_____
_____
_____
_____

MEAL 2 – TIME: _____

Most likely too many carbs	Balanced Responses
☐ Headache	☐ Appetite feels satisfied
☐ Anxiety	☐ Feel emotionally balanced
☐ Jittery/wired	☐ Good mental focus
☐ Difficulty concentrating	☐ Normal level of energy
☐ Hunger is not satisfied	☐ No cravings for sweets
☐ Crave sweet	☐ No cravings for more food
☐ Crave Protein & fat	

Most likely too much protein &/or fat

☐ Lethargic
☐ Mentally Sluggish
☐ Heavy Gut
☐ Feel full yet still hungry
☐ Crave sweets
☐ Crave Caffeine
(if more than hour after meal could be a crash from too much carb)

Approx. of macro Nutrient ratios of meal
% Carbs _____
% Protein _____
% Fat _____
Foods Eaten: _____
_____
_____
_____
_____

MEAL 3 – TIME: _____

Most likely too many carbs	Balanced Responses
☐ Headache	☐ Appetite feels satisfied
☐ Anxiety	☐ Feel emotionally balanced
☐ Jittery/wired	☐ Good mental focus
☐ Difficulty concentrating	☐ Normal level of energy
☐ Hunger is not satisfied	☐ No cravings for sweets
☐ Crave sweet	☐ No cravings for more food
☐ Crave Protein & fat	

Most likely too much protein &/or fat

☐ Lethargic
☐ Mentally Sluggish
☐ Heavy Gut
☐ Feel full yet still hungry
☐ Crave sweets
☐ Crave Caffeine
(if more than hour after meal could be a crash from too much carb)

Approx. of macro Nutrient ratios of meal
% Carbs _____
% Protein _____
% Fat _____
Foods Eaten: _____
_____
_____
_____
_____

SNACKS:

Time: _____ Details: _____
Time: _____ Details: _____
Time: _____ Details: _____

DRINKS:

Details: _____
_____
_____

LIFESTYLE:

What time did you go to sleep? _____ What time did you get up? _____
Sleep quality? ☐ Sound ☐ Restless   Did you have night Sweats? ☐ Yes ☐ No
Did you awake during night (give time & reason)? _____
Did you wake up refreshed today or tired? ☐ Refreshed ☐ Tired
Did you start slow this morning? ☐ Yes ☐ No   If yes, how long did it take to feel alert? _____

Bowel movement(s)?
(number, colour, size & shape)
_____
_____

MOVEMENT :

Details: _____
_____
_____

GENERAL:

How did you feel today? _____
_____
_____

OTHER INFO: _____

DAILY FOOD & LIFESTYLE DIARY

DAILY FOOD DIARY - DATE: _____

Complete everyday for 12 weeks

MEAL 1 – TIME: _____

Please fill out form 1-2 hours after each meal

Most likely too many carbs	Balanced Responses	Most likely too much protein &/or fat	
☐ Headache	☐ Appetite feels satisfied	☐ Lethargic	Approx. of macro Nutrient ratios of meal
☐ Anxiety	☐ Feel emotionally balanced	☐ Mentally Sluggish	% Carbs _____
☐ Jittery/wired	☐ Good mental focus	☐ Heavy Gut	% Protein _____
☐ Difficulty concentrating	☐ Normal level of energy	☐ Feel full yet still hungry	% Fat _____
☐ Hunger is not satisfied	☐ No cravings for sweets	☐ Crave sweets	Foods Eaten: _____
☐ Crave sweet	☐ No cravings for more food	☐ Crave Caffeine	_____
☐ Crave Protein & fat		(if more than hour after meal could	_____
		be a crash from too much carb)	_____
			_____
			_____

MEAL 2 – TIME: _____

Most likely too many carbs	Balanced Responses	Most likely too much protein &/or fat	
☐ Headache	☐ Appetite feels satisfied	☐ Lethargic	Approx. of macro Nutrient ratios of meal
☐ Anxiety	☐ Feel emotionally balanced	☐ Mentally Sluggish	% Carbs _____
☐ Jittery/wired	☐ Good mental focus	☐ Heavy Gut	% Protein _____
☐ Difficulty concentrating	☐ Normal level of energy	☐ Feel full yet still hungry	% Fat _____
☐ Hunger is not satisfied	☐ No cravings for sweets	☐ Crave sweets	Foods Eaten: _____
☐ Crave sweet	☐ No cravings for more food	☐ Crave Caffeine	_____
☐ Crave Protein & fat		(if more than hour after meal could	_____
		be a crash from too much carb)	_____
			_____
			_____

MEAL 3 – TIME: _____

Most likely too many carbs	Balanced Responses	Most likely too much protein &/or fat	
☐ Headache	☐ Appetite feels satisfied	☐ Lethargic	Approx. of macro Nutrient ratios of meal
☐ Anxiety	☐ Feel emotionally balanced	☐ Mentally Sluggish	% Carbs _____
☐ Jittery/wired	☐ Good mental focus	☐ Heavy Gut	% Protein _____
☐ Difficulty concentrating	☐ Normal level of energy	☐ Feel full yet still hungry	% Fat _____
☐ Hunger is not satisfied	☐ No cravings for sweets	☐ Crave sweets	Foods Eaten: _____
☐ Crave sweet	☐ No cravings for more food	☐ Crave Caffeine	_____
☐ Crave Protein & fat		(if more than hour after meal could	_____
		be a crash from too much carb)	_____
			_____
			_____

SNACKS:

Time: _____ Details: _____

Time: _____ Details: _____

Time: _____ Details: _____

DRINKS:

Details: _____

_____

_____

LIFESTYLE:

What time did you go to sleep? _____   What time did you get up? _____   Bowel movement(s)?

Sleep quality? ☐ Sound ☐ Restless   Did you have night Sweats? ☐ Yes ☐ No   (number, colour, size & shape)

Did you awake during night (give time & reason)? _____   _____

Did you wake up refreshed today or tired? ☐ Refreshed ☐ Tired   _____

Did you start slow this morning? ☐ Yes ☐ No   If yes, how long did it take to feel alert? _____

MOVEMENT :

Details: _____

_____

GENERAL:

How did you feel today? _____

_____

OTHER INFO: _____

181

DAILY FOOD & LIFESTYLE DIARY

DAILY FOOD DIARY - DATE: _____

MEAL 1 – TIME: _____

Complete everyday for 12 weeks

Please fill out form 1-2 hours after each meal

Most likely too many carbs	Balanced Responses	Most likely too much protein &/or fat	
☐ Headache	☐ Appetite feels satisfied	☐ Lethargic	Approx. of macro Nutrient ratios of meal
☐ Anxiety	☐ Feel emotionally balanced	☐ Mentally Sluggish	% Carbs _____
☐ Jittery/wired	☐ Good mental focus	☐ Heavy Gut	% Protein _____
☐ Difficulty concentrating	☐ Normal level of energy	☐ Feel full yet still hungry	% Fat _____
☐ Hunger is not satisfied	☐ No cravings for sweets	☐ Crave sweets	Foods Eaten: _____
☐ Crave sweet	☐ No cravings for more food	☐ Crave Caffeine	_____
☐ Crave Protein & fat		(if more than hour after meal could	_____
		be a crash from too much carb)	_____
			_____
			_____

MEAL 2 – TIME: _____

Most likely too many carbs	Balanced Responses	Most likely too much protein &/or fat	
☐ Headache	☐ Appetite feels satisfied	☐ Lethargic	Approx. of macro Nutrient ratios of meal
☐ Anxiety	☐ Feel emotionally balanced	☐ Mentally Sluggish	% Carbs _____
☐ Jittery/wired	☐ Good mental focus	☐ Heavy Gut	% Protein _____
☐ Difficulty concentrating	☐ Normal level of energy	☐ Feel full yet still hungry	% Fat _____
☐ Hunger is not satisfied	☐ No cravings for sweets	☐ Crave sweets	Foods Eaten: _____
☐ Crave sweet	☐ No cravings for more food	☐ Crave Caffeine	_____
☐ Crave Protein & fat		(if more than hour after meal could	_____
		be a crash from too much carb)	_____
			_____
			_____

MEAL 3 – TIME: _____

Most likely too many carbs	Balanced Responses	Most likely too much protein &/or fat	
☐ Headache	☐ Appetite feels satisfied	☐ Lethargic	Approx. of macro Nutrient ratios of meal
☐ Anxiety	☐ Feel emotionally balanced	☐ Mentally Sluggish	% Carbs _____
☐ Jittery/wired	☐ Good mental focus	☐ Heavy Gut	% Protein _____
☐ Difficulty concentrating	☐ Normal level of energy	☐ Feel full yet still hungry	% Fat _____
☐ Hunger is not satisfied	☐ No cravings for sweets	☐ Crave sweets	Foods Eaten: _____
☐ Crave sweet	☐ No cravings for more food	☐ Crave Caffeine	_____
☐ Crave Protein & fat		(if more than hour after meal could	_____
		be a crash from too much carb)	_____
			_____
			_____

SNACKS:

Time: _____ Details: _____

Time: _____ Details: _____

Time: _____ Details: _____

DRINKS:

Details: _____

_____

LIFESTYLE:

What time did you go to sleep? _____ What time did you get up? _____

Sleep quality? ☐ Sound ☐ Restless   Did you have night Sweats? ☐ Yes ☐ No

Did you awake during night (give time & reason)? _____

Did you wake up refreshed today or tired? ☐ Refreshed ☐ Tired

Did you start slow this morning? ☐ Yes ☐ No   If yes, how long did it take to feel alert? _____

Bowel movement(s)?

(number, colour, size & shape)

_____

_____

MOVEMENT :

Details: _____

_____

_____

GENERAL:

How did you feel today? _____

_____

_____

OTHER INFO: _____

DAILY FOOD & LIFESTYLE DIARY

DAILY FOOD DIARY - DATE: _____

Complete everyday for 12 weeks

MEAL 1 – TIME: _____

Please fill out form 1-2 hours after each meal

Most likely too many carbs	Balanced Responses	Most likely too much protein &/or fat	
☐ Headache	☐ Appetite feels satisfied	☐ Lethargic	Approx. of macro Nutrient ratios of meal
☐ Anxiety	☐ Feel emotionally balanced	☐ Mentally Sluggish	% Carbs _____
☐ Jittery/wired	☐ Good mental focus	☐ Heavy Gut	% Protein _____
☐ Difficulty concentrating	☐ Normal level of energy	☐ Feel full yet still hungry	% Fat _____
☐ Hunger is not satisfied	☐ No cravings for sweets	☐ Crave sweets	Foods Eaten: _____
☐ Crave sweet	☐ No cravings for more food	☐ Crave Caffeine	_____
☐ Crave Protein & fat		(if more than hour after meal could	_____
		be a crash from too much carb)	_____
			_____
			_____

MEAL 2 – TIME: _____

Most likely too many carbs	Balanced Responses	Most likely too much protein &/or fat	
☐ Headache	☐ Appetite feels satisfied	☐ Lethargic	Approx. of macro Nutrient ratios of meal
☐ Anxiety	☐ Feel emotionally balanced	☐ Mentally Sluggish	% Carbs _____
☐ Jittery/wired	☐ Good mental focus	☐ Heavy Gut	% Protein _____
☐ Difficulty concentrating	☐ Normal level of energy	☐ Feel full yet still hungry	% Fat _____
☐ Hunger is not satisfied	☐ No cravings for sweets	☐ Crave sweets	Foods Eaten: _____
☐ Crave sweet	☐ No cravings for more food	☐ Crave Caffeine	_____
☐ Crave Protein & fat		(if more than hour after meal could	_____
		be a crash from too much carb)	_____
			_____
			_____

MEAL 3 – TIME: _____

Most likely too many carbs	Balanced Responses	Most likely too much protein &/or fat	
☐ Headache	☐ Appetite feels satisfied	☐ Lethargic	Approx. of macro Nutrient ratios of meal
☐ Anxiety	☐ Feel emotionally balanced	☐ Mentally Sluggish	% Carbs _____
☐ Jittery/wired	☐ Good mental focus	☐ Heavy Gut	% Protein _____
☐ Difficulty concentrating	☐ Normal level of energy	☐ Feel full yet still hungry	% Fat _____
☐ Hunger is not satisfied	☐ No cravings for sweets	☐ Crave sweets	Foods Eaten: _____
☐ Crave sweet	☐ No cravings for more food	☐ Crave Caffeine	_____
☐ Crave Protein & fat		(if more than hour after meal could	_____
		be a crash from too much carb)	_____
			_____
			_____

SNACKS:

Time: _____ Details: _____

Time: _____ Details: _____

Time: _____ Details: _____

DRINKS:

Details: _____

_____

_____

LIFESTYLE:

What time did you go to sleep? _____ What time did you get up? _____

Sleep quality? ☐ Sound ☐ Restless Did you have night Sweats? ☐ Yes ☐ No

Did you awake during night (give time & reason)? _____

Did you wake up refreshed today or tired? ☐ Refreshed ☐ Tired

Did you start slow this morning? ☐ Yes ☐ No   If yes, how long did it take to feel alert? _____

Bowel movement(s)?
(number, colour, size & shape)

_____

_____

MOVEMENT :

Details: _____

_____

_____

GENERAL:

How did you feel today? _____

_____

OTHER INFO: _____

DAILY FOOD & LIFESTYLE DIARY

DAILY FOOD DIARY - DATE: _____

Complete everyday for 12 weeks

MEAL 1 – TIME: _____

Please fill out form 1-2 hours after each meal

Most likely too many carbs
- ☐ Headache
- ☐ Anxiety
- ☐ Jittery/wired
- ☐ Difficulty concentrating
- ☐ Hunger is not satisfied
- ☐ Crave sweet
- ☐ Crave Protein & fat

Balanced Responses
- ☐ Appetite feels satisfied
- ☐ Feel emotionally balanced
- ☐ Good mental focus
- ☐ Normal level of energy
- ☐ No cravings for sweets
- ☐ No cravings for more food

Most likely too much protein &/or fat
- ☐ Lethargic
- ☐ Mentally Sluggish
- ☐ Heavy Gut
- ☐ Feel full yet still hungry
- ☐ Crave sweets
- ☐ Crave Caffeine

(if more than hour after meal could be a crash from too much carb)

Approx. of macro Nutrient ratios of meal
% Carbs _____
% Protein _____
% Fat _____
Foods Eaten: _____
_____
_____
_____
_____

MEAL 2 – TIME: _____

Most likely too many carbs
- ☐ Headache
- ☐ Anxiety
- ☐ Jittery/wired
- ☐ Difficulty concentrating
- ☐ Hunger is not satisfied
- ☐ Crave sweet
- ☐ Crave Protein & fat

Balanced Responses
- ☐ Appetite feels satisfied
- ☐ Feel emotionally balanced
- ☐ Good mental focus
- ☐ Normal level of energy
- ☐ No cravings for sweets
- ☐ No cravings for more food

Most likely too much protein &/or fat
- ☐ Lethargic
- ☐ Mentally Sluggish
- ☐ Heavy Gut
- ☐ Feel full yet still hungry
- ☐ Crave sweets
- ☐ Crave Caffeine

(if more than hour after meal could be a crash from too much carb)

Approx. of macro Nutrient ratios of meal
% Carbs _____
% Protein _____
% Fat _____
Foods Eaten: _____
_____
_____
_____
_____

MEAL 3 – TIME: _____

Most likely too many carbs
- ☐ Headache
- ☐ Anxiety
- ☐ Jittery/wired
- ☐ Difficulty concentrating
- ☐ Hunger is not satisfied
- ☐ Crave sweet
- ☐ Crave Protein & fat

Balanced Responses
- ☐ Appetite feels satisfied
- ☐ Feel emotionally balanced
- ☐ Good mental focus
- ☐ Normal level of energy
- ☐ No cravings for sweets
- ☐ No cravings for more food

Most likely too much protein &/or fat
- ☐ Lethargic
- ☐ Mentally Sluggish
- ☐ Heavy Gut
- ☐ Feel full yet still hungry
- ☐ Crave sweets
- ☐ Crave Caffeine

(if more than hour after meal could be a crash from too much carb)

Approx. of macro Nutrient ratios of meal
% Carbs _____
% Protein _____
% Fat _____
Foods Eaten: _____
_____
_____
_____
_____

SNACKS:

Time: _____ Details: _____
Time: _____ Details: _____
Time: _____ Details: _____

DRINKS:

Details: _____
_____
_____

LIFESTYLE:

What time did you go to sleep?_____ What time did you get up? _____
Sleep quality? ☐ Sound ☐ Restless   Did you have night Sweats? ☐ Yes ☐ No
Did you awake during night (give time & reason)? _____
Did you wake up refreshed today or tired? ☐ Refreshed ☐ Tired
Did you start slow this morning? ☐ Yes ☐ No   If yes, how long did it take to feel alert? _____

Bowel movement(s)?
(number, colour, size & shape)
_____
_____

MOVEMENT :

Details:_____
_____
_____

GENERAL:

How did you feel today? _____
_____
_____

OTHER INFO: _____

DAILY FOOD & LIFESTYLE DIARY

DAILY FOOD DIARY - DATE: _____

Complete everyday for 12 weeks

MEAL 1 – TIME: _____

Please fill out form 1-2 hours after each meal

Most likely too many carbs

- ☐ Headache
- ☐ Anxiety
- ☐ Jittery/wired
- ☐ Difficulty concentrating
- ☐ Hunger is not satisfied
- ☐ Crave sweet
- ☐ Crave Protein & fat

Balanced Responses

- ☐ Appetite feels satisfied
- ☐ Feel emotionally balanced
- ☐ Good mental focus
- ☐ Normal level of energy
- ☐ No cravings for sweets
- ☐ No cravings for more food

Most likely too much protein &/or fat

- ☐ Lethargic
- ☐ Mentally Sluggish
- ☐ Heavy Gut
- ☐ Feel full yet still hungry
- ☐ Crave sweets
- ☐ Crave Caffeine

(if more than hour after meal could be a crash from too much carb)

Approx. of macro Nutrient ratios of meal

% Carbs _____
% Protein _____
% Fat _____
Foods Eaten: _____
_____
_____
_____
_____
_____

MEAL 2 – TIME: _____

Most likely too many carbs

- ☐ Headache
- ☐ Anxiety
- ☐ Jittery/wired
- ☐ Difficulty concentrating
- ☐ Hunger is not satisfied
- ☐ Crave sweet
- ☐ Crave Protein & fat

Balanced Responses

- ☐ Appetite feels satisfied
- ☐ Feel emotionally balanced
- ☐ Good mental focus
- ☐ Normal level of energy
- ☐ No cravings for sweets
- ☐ No cravings for more food

Most likely too much protein &/or fat

- ☐ Lethargic
- ☐ Mentally Sluggish
- ☐ Heavy Gut
- ☐ Feel full yet still hungry
- ☐ Crave sweets
- ☐ Crave Caffeine

(if more than hour after meal could be a crash from too much carb)

Approx. of macro Nutrient ratios of meal

% Carbs _____
% Protein _____
% Fat _____
Foods Eaten: _____
_____
_____
_____
_____

MEAL 3 – TIME: _____

Most likely too many carbs

- ☐ Headache
- ☐ Anxiety
- ☐ Jittery/wired
- ☐ Difficulty concentrating
- ☐ Hunger is not satisfied
- ☐ Crave sweet
- ☐ Crave Protein & fat

Balanced Responses

- ☐ Appetite feels satisfied
- ☐ Feel emotionally balanced
- ☐ Good mental focus
- ☐ Normal level of energy
- ☐ No cravings for sweets
- ☐ No cravings for more food

Most likely too much protein &/or fat

- ☐ Lethargic
- ☐ Mentally Sluggish
- ☐ Heavy Gut
- ☐ Feel full yet still hungry
- ☐ Crave sweets
- ☐ Crave Caffeine

(if more than hour after meal could be a crash from too much carb)

Approx. of macro Nutrient ratios of meal

% Carbs _____
% Protein _____
% Fat _____
Foods Eaten: _____
_____
_____
_____
_____

SNACKS:

Time: _____ Details: _____
Time: _____ Details: _____
Time: _____ Details: _____

DRINKS:

Details: _____
_____
_____

LIFESTYLE:

What time did you go to sleep? _____ What time did you get up? _____

Sleep quality? ☐ Sound ☐ Restless Did you have night Sweats? ☐ Yes ☐ No

Did you awake during night (give time & reason)? _____

Did you wake up refreshed today or tired? ☐ Refreshed ☐ Tired

Did you start slow this morning? ☐ Yes ☐ No If yes, how long did it take to feel alert? _____

Bowel movement(s)?
(number, colour, size & shape)
_____
_____

MOVEMENT :

Details: _____
_____
_____

GENERAL:

How did you feel today? _____
_____

OTHER INFO: _____

185

DAILY FOOD & LIFESTYLE DIARY

DAILY FOOD DIARY - DATE: _____

Complete everyday for 12 weeks

MEAL 1 – TIME: _____

Please fill out form 1-2 hours after each meal

Most likely too many carbs	Balanced Responses	Most likely too much protein &/or fat	
☐ Headache	☐ Appetite feels satisfied	☐ Lethargic	Approx. of macro Nutrient ratios of meal
☐ Anxiety	☐ Feel emotionally balanced	☐ Mentally Sluggish	% Carbs _____
☐ Jittery/wired	☐ Good mental focus	☐ Heavy Gut	% Protein _____
☐ Difficulty concentrating	☐ Normal level of energy	☐ Feel full yet still hungry	% Fat _____
☐ Hunger is not satisfied	☐ No cravings for sweets	☐ Crave sweets	Foods Eaten: _____
☐ Crave sweet	☐ No cravings for more food	☐ Crave Caffeine	_____
☐ Crave Protein & fat		(if more than hour after meal could	_____
		be a crash from too much carb)	_____

MEAL 2 – TIME: _____

Most likely too many carbs	Balanced Responses	Most likely too much protein &/or fat	
☐ Headache	☐ Appetite feels satisfied	☐ Lethargic	Approx. of macro Nutrient ratios of meal
☐ Anxiety	☐ Feel emotionally balanced	☐ Mentally Sluggish	% Carbs _____
☐ Jittery/wired	☐ Good mental focus	☐ Heavy Gut	% Protein _____
☐ Difficulty concentrating	☐ Normal level of energy	☐ Feel full yet still hungry	% Fat _____
☐ Hunger is not satisfied	☐ No cravings for sweets	☐ Crave sweets	Foods Eaten: _____
☐ Crave sweet	☐ No cravings for more food	☐ Crave Caffeine	_____
☐ Crave Protein & fat		(if more than hour after meal could	_____
		be a crash from too much carb)	_____

MEAL 3 – TIME: _____

Most likely too many carbs	Balanced Responses	Most likely too much protein &/or fat	
☐ Headache	☐ Appetite feels satisfied	☐ Lethargic	Approx. of macro Nutrient ratios of meal
☐ Anxiety	☐ Feel emotionally balanced	☐ Mentally Sluggish	% Carbs _____
☐ Jittery/wired	☐ Good mental focus	☐ Heavy Gut	% Protein _____
☐ Difficulty concentrating	☐ Normal level of energy	☐ Feel full yet still hungry	% Fat _____
☐ Hunger is not satisfied	☐ No cravings for sweets	☐ Crave sweets	Foods Eaten: _____
☐ Crave sweet	☐ No cravings for more food	☐ Crave Caffeine	_____
☐ Crave Protein & fat		(if more than hour after meal could	_____
		be a crash from too much carb)	_____

SNACKS:

Time: _____ Details: _____

Time: _____ Details: _____

Time: _____ Details: _____

DRINKS:

Details: _____

_____

LIFESTYLE:

What time did you go to sleep?_____ What time did you get up? _____

Sleep quality? ☐ Sound ☐ Restless   Did you have night Sweats? ☐ Yes ☐ No

Did you awake during night (give time & reason)? _____

Did you wake up refreshed today or tired? ☐ Refreshed ☐ Tired

Did you start slow this morning? ☐ Yes ☐ No   If yes, how long did it take to feel alert? _____

Bowel movement(s)?
(number, colour, size & shape)

_____

_____

MOVEMENT :

Details: _____

_____

GENERAL:

How did you feel today? _____

_____

OTHER INFO: _____

DAILY FOOD & LIFESTYLE DIARY

DAILY FOOD DIARY - DATE: _____

MEAL 1 – TIME: _____

Complete everyday for 12 weeks

Please fill out form 1-2 hours after each meal

Most likely too many carbs

- ☐ Headache
- ☐ Anxiety
- ☐ Jittery/wired
- ☐ Difficulty concentrating
- ☐ Hunger is not satisfied
- ☐ Crave sweet
- ☐ Crave Protein & fat

Balanced Responses

- ☐ Appetite feels satisfied
- ☐ Feel emotionally balanced
- ☐ Good mental focus
- ☐ Normal level of energy
- ☐ No cravings for sweets
- ☐ No cravings for more food

Most likely too much protein &/or fat

- ☐ Lethargic
- ☐ Mentally Sluggish
- ☐ Heavy Gut
- ☐ Feel full yet still hungry
- ☐ Crave sweets
- ☐ Crave Caffeine

(if more than hour after meal could be a crash from too much carb)

Approx. of macro Nutrient ratios of meal

% Carbs _____
% Protein _____
% Fat _____

Foods Eaten: _____
_____
_____
_____
_____
_____

MEAL 2 – TIME: _____

Most likely too many carbs

- ☐ Headache
- ☐ Anxiety
- ☐ Jittery/wired
- ☐ Difficulty concentrating
- ☐ Hunger is not satisfied
- ☐ Crave sweet
- ☐ Crave Protein & fat

Balanced Responses

- ☐ Appetite feels satisfied
- ☐ Feel emotionally balanced
- ☐ Good mental focus
- ☐ Normal level of energy
- ☐ No cravings for sweets
- ☐ No cravings for more food

Most likely too much protein &/or fat

- ☐ Lethargic
- ☐ Mentally Sluggish
- ☐ Heavy Gut
- ☐ Feel full yet still hungry
- ☐ Crave sweets
- ☐ Crave Caffeine

(if more than hour after meal could be a crash from too much carb)

Approx. of macro Nutrient ratios of meal

% Carbs _____
% Protein _____
% Fat _____

Foods Eaten: _____
_____
_____
_____
_____
_____

MEAL 3 – TIME: _____

Most likely too many carbs

- ☐ Headache
- ☐ Anxiety
- ☐ Jittery/wired
- ☐ Difficulty concentrating
- ☐ Hunger is not satisfied
- ☐ Crave sweet
- ☐ Crave Protein & fat

Balanced Responses

- ☐ Appetite feels satisfied
- ☐ Feel emotionally balanced
- ☐ Good mental focus
- ☐ Normal level of energy
- ☐ No cravings for sweets
- ☐ No cravings for more food

Most likely too much protein &/or fat

- ☐ Lethargic
- ☐ Mentally Sluggish
- ☐ Heavy Gut
- ☐ Feel full yet still hungry
- ☐ Crave sweets
- ☐ Crave Caffeine

(if more than hour after meal could be a crash from too much carb)

Approx. of macro Nutrient ratios of meal

% Carbs _____
% Protein _____
% Fat _____

Foods Eaten: _____
_____
_____
_____
_____
_____

SNACKS:

Time: _____ Details: _____
Time: _____ Details: _____
Time: _____ Details: _____

DRINKS:

Details: _____
_____
_____

LIFESTYLE:

What time did you go to sleep? _____ What time did you get up? _____
Sleep quality? ☐ Sound ☐ Restless   Did you have night Sweats? ☐ Yes ☐ No
Did you awake during night (give time & reason)? _____
Did you wake up refreshed today or tired? ☐ Refreshed ☐ Tired
Did you start slow this morning? ☐ Yes ☐ No   If yes, how long did it take to feel alert? _____

Bowel movement(s)?
(number, colour, size & shape)
_____
_____

MOVEMENT :

Details: _____
_____
_____

GENERAL:

How did you feel today? _____
_____
_____

OTHER INFO: _____

DAILY FOOD & LIFESTYLE DIARY

DAILY FOOD DIARY - DATE: _____

Complete everyday for 12 weeks

MEAL 1 – TIME: _____

Please fill out form 1-2 hours after each meal

Most likely too many carbs	Balanced Responses	Most likely too much protein &/or fat	Approx. of macro Nutrient ratios of meal
☐ Headache	☐ Appetite feels satisfied	☐ Lethargic	% Carbs _____
☐ Anxiety	☐ Feel emotionally balanced	☐ Mentally Sluggish	% Protein _____
☐ Jittery/wired	☐ Good mental focus	☐ Heavy Gut	% Fat _____
☐ Difficulty concentrating	☐ Normal level of energy	☐ Feel full yet still hungry	Foods Eaten: _____
☐ Hunger is not satisfied	☐ No cravings for sweets	☐ Crave sweets	
☐ Crave sweet	☐ No cravings for more food	☐ Crave Caffeine	
☐ Crave Protein & fat		(if more than hour after meal could be a crash from too much carb)	

MEAL 2 – TIME: _____

Most likely too many carbs	Balanced Responses	Most likely too much protein &/or fat	Approx. of macro Nutrient ratios of meal
☐ Headache	☐ Appetite feels satisfied	☐ Lethargic	% Carbs _____
☐ Anxiety	☐ Feel emotionally balanced	☐ Mentally Sluggish	% Protein _____
☐ Jittery/wired	☐ Good mental focus	☐ Heavy Gut	% Fat _____
☐ Difficulty concentrating	☐ Normal level of energy	☐ Feel full yet still hungry	Foods Eaten: _____
☐ Hunger is not satisfied	☐ No cravings for sweets	☐ Crave sweets	
☐ Crave sweet	☐ No cravings for more food	☐ Crave Caffeine	
☐ Crave Protein & fat		(if more than hour after meal could be a crash from too much carb)	

MEAL 3 – TIME: _____

Most likely too many carbs	Balanced Responses	Most likely too much protein &/or fat	Approx. of macro Nutrient ratios of meal
☐ Headache	☐ Appetite feels satisfied	☐ Lethargic	% Carbs _____
☐ Anxiety	☐ Feel emotionally balanced	☐ Mentally Sluggish	% Protein _____
☐ Jittery/wired	☐ Good mental focus	☐ Heavy Gut	% Fat _____
☐ Difficulty concentrating	☐ Normal level of energy	☐ Feel full yet still hungry	Foods Eaten: _____
☐ Hunger is not satisfied	☐ No cravings for sweets	☐ Crave sweets	
☐ Crave sweet	☐ No cravings for more food	☐ Crave Caffeine	
☐ Crave Protein & fat		(if more than hour after meal could be a crash from too much carb)	

SNACKS:

Time: _____ Details: _____
Time: _____ Details: _____
Time: _____ Details: _____

DRINKS:

Details: _____

LIFESTYLE:

What time did you go to sleep?_____ What time did you get up? _____ Bowel movement(s)?
Sleep quality? ☐ Sound ☐ Restless   Did you have night Sweats? ☐ Yes ☐ No   (number, colour, size & shape)
Did you awake during night (give time & reason)? _____
Did you wake up refreshed today or tired? ☐ Refreshed ☐ Tired
Did you start slow this morning? ☐ Yes ☐ No   If yes, how long did it take to feel alert? _____

MOVEMENT :

Details: _____

GENERAL:

How did you feel today? _____

OTHER INFO: _____

DAILY FOOD & LIFESTYLE DIARY

DAILY FOOD DIARY - DATE: _____

Complete everyday for 12 weeks

MEAL 1 – TIME: _____

Please fill out form 1-2 hours after each meal

Most likely too many carbs

- ☐ Headache
- ☐ Anxiety
- ☐ Jittery/wired
- ☐ Difficulty concentrating
- ☐ Hunger is not satisfied
- ☐ Crave sweet
- ☐ Crave Protein & fat

Balanced Responses

- ☐ Appetite feels satisfied
- ☐ Feel emotionally balanced
- ☐ Good mental focus
- ☐ Normal level of energy
- ☐ No cravings for sweets
- ☐ No cravings for more food

Most likely too much protein &/or fat

- ☐ Lethargic
- ☐ Mentally Sluggish
- ☐ Heavy Gut
- ☐ Feel full yet still hungry
- ☐ Crave sweets
- ☐ Crave Caffeine
(if more than hour after meal could be a crash from too much carb)

Approx. of macro Nutrient ratios of meal
% Carbs _____
% Protein _____
% Fat _____
Foods Eaten: _____
_____
_____
_____
_____
_____

MEAL 2 – TIME: _____

Most likely too many carbs

- ☐ Headache
- ☐ Anxiety
- ☐ Jittery/wired
- ☐ Difficulty concentrating
- ☐ Hunger is not satisfied
- ☐ Crave sweet
- ☐ Crave Protein & fat

Balanced Responses

- ☐ Appetite feels satisfied
- ☐ Feel emotionally balanced
- ☐ Good mental focus
- ☐ Normal level of energy
- ☐ No cravings for sweets
- ☐ No cravings for more food

Most likely too much protein &/or fat

- ☐ Lethargic
- ☐ Mentally Sluggish
- ☐ Heavy Gut
- ☐ Feel full yet still hungry
- ☐ Crave sweets
- ☐ Crave Caffeine
(if more than hour after meal could be a crash from too much carb)

Approx. of macro Nutrient ratios of meal
% Carbs _____
% Protein _____
% Fat _____
Foods Eaten: _____
_____
_____
_____
_____
_____

MEAL 3 – TIME: _____

Most likely too many carbs

- ☐ Headache
- ☐ Anxiety
- ☐ Jittery/wired
- ☐ Difficulty concentrating
- ☐ Hunger is not satisfied
- ☐ Crave sweet
- ☐ Crave Protein & fat

Balanced Responses

- ☐ Appetite feels satisfied
- ☐ Feel emotionally balanced
- ☐ Good mental focus
- ☐ Normal level of energy
- ☐ No cravings for sweets
- ☐ No cravings for more food

Most likely too much protein &/or fat

- ☐ Lethargic
- ☐ Mentally Sluggish
- ☐ Heavy Gut
- ☐ Feel full yet still hungry
- ☐ Crave sweets
- ☐ Crave Caffeine
(if more than hour after meal could be a crash from too much carb)

Approx. of macro Nutrient ratios of meal
% Carbs _____
% Protein _____
% Fat _____
Foods Eaten: _____
_____
_____
_____
_____
_____

SNACKS:

Time: _____ Details: _____
Time: _____ Details: _____
Time: _____ Details: _____

DRINKS:

Details: _____
_____
_____

LIFESTYLE:

What time did you go to sleep? _____ What time did you get up? _____
Sleep quality? ☐ Sound ☐ Restless   Did you have night Sweats? ☐ Yes ☐ No
Did you awake during night (give time & reason)? _____
Did you wake up refreshed today or tired? ☐ Refreshed ☐ Tired
Did you start slow this morning? ☐ Yes ☐ No   If yes, how long did it take to feel alert? _____

Bowel movement(s)?
(number, colour, size & shape)
_____
_____

MOVEMENT :

Details: _____
_____
_____

GENERAL:

How did you feel today? _____
_____
_____

OTHER INFO: _____

DAILY FOOD & LIFESTYLE DIARY

DAILY FOOD DIARY - DATE: _____

MEAL 1 – TIME: _____

Complete everyday for 12 weeks

Please fill out form 1-2 hours after each meal

Most likely too many carbs	Balanced Responses	Most likely too much protein &/or fat	
☐ Headache	☐ Appetite feels satisfied	☐ Lethargic	Approx. of macro Nutrient ratios of meal
☐ Anxiety	☐ Feel emotionally balanced	☐ Mentally Sluggish	% Carbs _____
☐ Jittery/wired	☐ Good mental focus	☐ Heavy Gut	% Protein _____
☐ Difficulty concentrating	☐ Normal level of energy	☐ Feel full yet still hungry	% Fat _____
☐ Hunger is not satisfied	☐ No cravings for sweets	☐ Crave sweets	Foods Eaten: _____
☐ Crave sweet	☐ No cravings for more food	☐ Crave Caffeine	_____
☐ Crave Protein & fat		(if more than hour after meal could be a crash from too much carb)	_____

MEAL 2 – TIME: _____

Most likely too many carbs	Balanced Responses	Most likely too much protein &/or fat	
☐ Headache	☐ Appetite feels satisfied	☐ Lethargic	Approx. of macro Nutrient ratios of meal
☐ Anxiety	☐ Feel emotionally balanced	☐ Mentally Sluggish	% Carbs _____
☐ Jittery/wired	☐ Good mental focus	☐ Heavy Gut	% Protein _____
☐ Difficulty concentrating	☐ Normal level of energy	☐ Feel full yet still hungry	% Fat _____
☐ Hunger is not satisfied	☐ No cravings for sweets	☐ Crave sweets	Foods Eaten: _____
☐ Crave sweet	☐ No cravings for more food	☐ Crave Caffeine	_____
☐ Crave Protein & fat		(if more than hour after meal could be a crash from too much carb)	_____

MEAL 3 – TIME: _____

Most likely too many carbs	Balanced Responses	Most likely too much protein &/or fat	
☐ Headache	☐ Appetite feels satisfied	☐ Lethargic	Approx. of macro Nutrient ratios of meal
☐ Anxiety	☐ Feel emotionally balanced	☐ Mentally Sluggish	% Carbs _____
☐ Jittery/wired	☐ Good mental focus	☐ Heavy Gut	% Protein _____
☐ Difficulty concentrating	☐ Normal level of energy	☐ Feel full yet still hungry	% Fat _____
☐ Hunger is not satisfied	☐ No cravings for sweets	☐ Crave sweets	Foods Eaten: _____
☐ Crave sweet	☐ No cravings for more food	☐ Crave Caffeine	_____
☐ Crave Protein & fat		(if more than hour after meal could be a crash from too much carb)	_____

SNACKS:

Time: _____ Details: _____
Time: _____ Details: _____
Time: _____ Details: _____

DRINKS:

Details: _____
_____
_____

LIFESTYLE:

What time did you go to sleep?_____ What time did you get up? _____
Sleep quality? ☐ Sound ☐ Restless   Did you have night Sweats? ☐ Yes ☐ No
Did you awake during night (give time & reason)? _____
Did you wake up refreshed today or tired? ☐ Refreshed ☐ Tired
Did you start slow this morning? ☐ Yes ☐ No   If yes, how long did it take to feel alert? _____

Bowel movement(s)?
(number, colour, size & shape)
_____
_____

MOVEMENT :

Details: _____
_____
_____

GENERAL:

How did you feel today? _____
_____
_____

OTHER INFO: _____

DAILY FOOD & LIFESTYLE DIARY

DAILY FOOD DIARY - DATE: _____   Complete everyday for 12 weeks

MEAL 1 – TIME: _____   Please fill out form 1-2 hours after each meal

Most likely too many carbs	Balanced Responses	Most likely too much protein &/or fat
☐ Headache	☐ Appetite feels satisfied	☐ Lethargic
☐ Anxiety	☐ Feel emotionally balanced	☐ Mentally Sluggish
☐ Jittery/wired	☐ Good mental focus	☐ Heavy Gut
☐ Difficulty concentrating	☐ Normal level of energy	☐ Feel full yet still hungry
☐ Hunger is not satisfied	☐ No cravings for sweets	☐ Crave sweets
☐ Crave sweet	☐ No cravings for more food	☐ Crave Caffeine
☐ Crave Protein & fat		(if more than hour after meal could be a crash from too much carb)

Approx. of macro Nutrient ratios of meal
% Carbs _____
% Protein _____
% Fat _____
Foods Eaten: _____
_____
_____
_____
_____
_____

MEAL 2 – TIME: _____

Most likely too many carbs	Balanced Responses	Most likely too much protein &/or fat
☐ Headache	☐ Appetite feels satisfied	☐ Lethargic
☐ Anxiety	☐ Feel emotionally balanced	☐ Mentally Sluggish
☐ Jittery/wired	☐ Good mental focus	☐ Heavy Gut
☐ Difficulty concentrating	☐ Normal level of energy	☐ Feel full yet still hungry
☐ Hunger is not satisfied	☐ No cravings for sweets	☐ Crave sweets
☐ Crave sweet	☐ No cravings for more food	☐ Crave Caffeine
☐ Crave Protein & fat		(if more than hour after meal could be a crash from too much carb)

Approx. of macro Nutrient ratios of meal
% Carbs _____
% Protein _____
% Fat _____
Foods Eaten: _____
_____
_____
_____
_____
_____

MEAL 3 – TIME: _____

Most likely too many carbs	Balanced Responses	Most likely too much protein &/or fat
☐ Headache	☐ Appetite feels satisfied	☐ Lethargic
☐ Anxiety	☐ Feel emotionally balanced	☐ Mentally Sluggish
☐ Jittery/wired	☐ Good mental focus	☐ Heavy Gut
☐ Difficulty concentrating	☐ Normal level of energy	☐ Feel full yet still hungry
☐ Hunger is not satisfied	☐ No cravings for sweets	☐ Crave sweets
☐ Crave sweet	☐ No cravings for more food	☐ Crave Caffeine
☐ Crave Protein & fat		(if more than hour after meal could be a crash from too much carb)

Approx. of macro Nutrient ratios of meal
% Carbs _____
% Protein _____
% Fat _____
Foods Eaten: _____
_____
_____
_____
_____
_____

SNACKS:

Time: _____ Details: _____
Time: _____ Details: _____
Time: _____ Details: _____

DRINKS:

Details: _____
_____
_____

LIFESTYLE:

What time did you go to sleep? _____ What time did you get up? _____
Sleep quality? ☐ Sound ☐ Restless   Did you have night Sweats? ☐ Yes ☐ No
Did you awake during night (give time & reason)? _____
Did you wake up refreshed today or tired? ☐ Refreshed ☐ Tired
Did you start slow this morning? ☐ Yes ☐ No   If yes, how long did it take to feel alert? _____

Bowel movement(s)?
(number, colour, size & shape)
_____
_____

MOVEMENT :

Details: _____
_____

GENERAL:

How did you feel today? _____
_____

OTHER INFO: _____

DAILY FOOD & LIFESTYLE DIARY

DAILY FOOD DIARY - DATE: _____

Complete everyday for 12 weeks

MEAL 1 – TIME: _____

Please fill out form 1-2 hours after each meal

Most likely too many carbs	Balanced Responses	Most likely too much protein &/or fat	
☐ Headache	☐ Appetite feels satisfied	☐ Lethargic	Approx. of macro Nutrient ratios of meal
☐ Anxiety	☐ Feel emotionally balanced	☐ Mentally Sluggish	% Carbs _____
☐ Jittery/wired	☐ Good mental focus	☐ Heavy Gut	% Protein _____
☐ Difficulty concentrating	☐ Normal level of energy	☐ Feel full yet still hungry	% Fat _____
☐ Hunger is not satisfied	☐ No cravings for sweets	☐ Crave sweets	Foods Eaten: _____
☐ Crave sweet	☐ No cravings for more food	☐ Crave Caffeine	_____
☐ Crave Protein & fat		(if more than hour after meal could be a crash from too much carb)	_____ _____ _____ _____

MEAL 2 – TIME: _____

Most likely too many carbs	Balanced Responses	Most likely too much protein &/or fat	
☐ Headache	☐ Appetite feels satisfied	☐ Lethargic	Approx. of macro Nutrient ratios of meal
☐ Anxiety	☐ Feel emotionally balanced	☐ Mentally Sluggish	% Carbs _____
☐ Jittery/wired	☐ Good mental focus	☐ Heavy Gut	% Protein _____
☐ Difficulty concentrating	☐ Normal level of energy	☐ Feel full yet still hungry	% Fat _____
☐ Hunger is not satisfied	☐ No cravings for sweets	☐ Crave sweets	Foods Eaten: _____
☐ Crave sweet	☐ No cravings for more food	☐ Crave Caffeine	_____
☐ Crave Protein & fat		(if more than hour after meal could be a crash from too much carb)	_____ _____ _____ _____

MEAL 3 – TIME: _____

Most likely too many carbs	Balanced Responses	Most likely too much protein &/or fat	
☐ Headache	☐ Appetite feels satisfied	☐ Lethargic	Approx. of macro Nutrient ratios of meal
☐ Anxiety	☐ Feel emotionally balanced	☐ Mentally Sluggish	% Carbs _____
☐ Jittery/wired	☐ Good mental focus	☐ Heavy Gut	% Protein _____
☐ Difficulty concentrating	☐ Normal level of energy	☐ Feel full yet still hungry	% Fat _____
☐ Hunger is not satisfied	☐ No cravings for sweets	☐ Crave sweets	Foods Eaten: _____
☐ Crave sweet	☐ No cravings for more food	☐ Crave Caffeine	_____
☐ Crave Protein & fat		(if more than hour after meal could be a crash from too much carb)	_____ _____ _____ _____

SNACKS:

Time: _____ Details: _____
Time: _____ Details: _____
Time: _____ Details: _____

DRINKS:

Details: _____
_____
_____

LIFESTYLE:

What time did you go to sleep? _____ What time did you get up? _____ Bowel movement(s)?
Sleep quality? ☐ Sound ☐ Restless   Did you have night Sweats? ☐ Yes ☐ No   (number, colour, size & shape)
Did you awake during night (give time & reason)? _____
Did you wake up refreshed today or tired? ☐ Refreshed ☐ Tired
Did you start slow this morning? ☐ Yes ☐ No   If yes, how long did it take to feel alert? _____

MOVEMENT :

Details: _____
_____
_____

GENERAL:

How did you feel today? _____
_____

OTHER INFO: _____

DAILY FOOD & LIFESTYLE DIARY

DAILY FOOD DIARY - DATE: _____

Complete everyday for 12 weeks

MEAL 1 – TIME: _____

Please fill out form 1-2 hours after each meal

Most likely too many carbs	Balanced Responses	Most likely too much protein &/or fat	
☐ Headache	☐ Appetite feels satisfied	☐ Lethargic	Approx. of macro Nutrient ratios of meal
☐ Anxiety	☐ Feel emotionally balanced	☐ Mentally Sluggish	% Carbs _____
☐ Jittery/wired	☐ Good mental focus	☐ Heavy Gut	% Protein _____
☐ Difficulty concentrating	☐ Normal level of energy	☐ Feel full yet still hungry	% Fat _____
☐ Hunger is not satisfied	☐ No cravings for sweets	☐ Crave sweets	Foods Eaten: _____
☐ Crave sweet	☐ No cravings for more food	☐ Crave Caffeine	_____
☐ Crave Protein & fat		(if more than hour after meal could	_____
		be a crash from too much carb)	_____
			_____
			_____

MEAL 2 – TIME: _____

Most likely too many carbs	Balanced Responses	Most likely too much protein &/or fat	
☐ Headache	☐ Appetite feels satisfied	☐ Lethargic	Approx. of macro Nutrient ratios of meal
☐ Anxiety	☐ Feel emotionally balanced	☐ Mentally Sluggish	% Carbs _____
☐ Jittery/wired	☐ Good mental focus	☐ Heavy Gut	% Protein _____
☐ Difficulty concentrating	☐ Normal level of energy	☐ Feel full yet still hungry	% Fat _____
☐ Hunger is not satisfied	☐ No cravings for sweets	☐ Crave sweets	Foods Eaten: _____
☐ Crave sweet	☐ No cravings for more food	☐ Crave Caffeine	_____
☐ Crave Protein & fat		(if more than hour after meal could	_____
		be a crash from too much carb)	_____
			_____
			_____

MEAL 3 – TIME: _____

Most likely too many carbs	Balanced Responses	Most likely too much protein &/or fat	
☐ Headache	☐ Appetite feels satisfied	☐ Lethargic	Approx. of macro Nutrient ratios of meal
☐ Anxiety	☐ Feel emotionally balanced	☐ Mentally Sluggish	% Carbs _____
☐ Jittery/wired	☐ Good mental focus	☐ Heavy Gut	% Protein _____
☐ Difficulty concentrating	☐ Normal level of energy	☐ Feel full yet still hungry	% Fat _____
☐ Hunger is not satisfied	☐ No cravings for sweets	☐ Crave sweets	Foods Eaten: _____
☐ Crave sweet	☐ No cravings for more food	☐ Crave Caffeine	_____
☐ Crave Protein & fat		(if more than hour after meal could	_____
		be a crash from too much carb)	_____
			_____
			_____

SNACKS:

Time: _____ Details: _____

Time: _____ Details: _____

Time: _____ Details: _____

DRINKS:

Details: _____

_____

LIFESTYLE:

What time did you go to sleep?_____ What time did you get up? _____ Bowel movement(s)?

Sleep quality? ☐ Sound ☐ Restless   Did you have night Sweats? ☐ Yes ☐ No   (number, colour, size & shape)

Did you awake during night (give time & reason)? _____ _____

Did you wake up refreshed today or tired? ☐ Refreshed ☐ Tired   _____

Did you start slow this morning? ☐ Yes ☐ No   If yes, how long did it take to feel alert? _____

MOVEMENT :

Details: _____

_____

_____

GENERAL:

How did you feel today? _____

_____

_____

OTHER INFO: _____

DAILY FOOD & LIFESTYLE DIARY

DAILY FOOD DIARY - DATE: _____

Complete everyday for 12 weeks

MEAL 1 – TIME: _____

Please fill out form 1-2 hours after each meal

Most likely too many carbs	Balanced Responses	Most likely too much protein &/or fat	
☐ Headache	☐ Appetite feels satisfied	☐ Lethargic	Approx. of macro Nutrient ratios of meal
☐ Anxiety	☐ Feel emotionally balanced	☐ Mentally Sluggish	% Carbs _____
☐ Jittery/wired	☐ Good mental focus	☐ Heavy Gut	% Protein _____
☐ Difficulty concentrating	☐ Normal level of energy	☐ Feel full yet still hungry	% Fat _____
☐ Hunger is not satisfied	☐ No cravings for sweets	☐ Crave sweets	Foods Eaten: _____
☐ Crave sweet	☐ No cravings for more food	☐ Crave Caffeine	_____
☐ Crave Protein & fat		(if more than hour after meal could	_____
		be a crash from too much carb)	_____
			_____
			_____

MEAL 2 – TIME: _____

Most likely too many carbs	Balanced Responses	Most likely too much protein &/or fat	
☐ Headache	☐ Appetite feels satisfied	☐ Lethargic	Approx. of macro Nutrient ratios of meal
☐ Anxiety	☐ Feel emotionally balanced	☐ Mentally Sluggish	% Carbs _____
☐ Jittery/wired	☐ Good mental focus	☐ Heavy Gut	% Protein _____
☐ Difficulty concentrating	☐ Normal level of energy	☐ Feel full yet still hungry	% Fat _____
☐ Hunger is not satisfied	☐ No cravings for sweets	☐ Crave sweets	Foods Eaten: _____
☐ Crave sweet	☐ No cravings for more food	☐ Crave Caffeine	_____
☐ Crave Protein & fat		(if more than hour after meal could	_____
		be a crash from too much carb)	_____
			_____
			_____

MEAL 3 – TIME: _____

Most likely too many carbs	Balanced Responses	Most likely too much protein &/or fat	
☐ Headache	☐ Appetite feels satisfied	☐ Lethargic	Approx. of macro Nutrient ratios of meal
☐ Anxiety	☐ Feel emotionally balanced	☐ Mentally Sluggish	% Carbs _____
☐ Jittery/wired	☐ Good mental focus	☐ Heavy Gut	% Protein _____
☐ Difficulty concentrating	☐ Normal level of energy	☐ Feel full yet still hungry	% Fat _____
☐ Hunger is not satisfied	☐ No cravings for sweets	☐ Crave sweets	Foods Eaten: _____
☐ Crave sweet	☐ No cravings for more food	☐ Crave Caffeine	_____
☐ Crave Protein & fat		(if more than hour after meal could	_____
		be a crash from too much carb)	_____
			_____
			_____

SNACKS:

Time: _____ Details: _____

Time: _____ Details: _____

Time: _____ Details: _____

DRINKS:

Details: _____

_____

_____

LIFESTYLE:

What time did you go to sleep? _____   What time did you get up? _____   Bowel movement(s)?

Sleep quality? ☐ Sound ☐ Restless   Did you have night Sweats? ☐ Yes ☐ No   (number, colour, size & shape)

Did you awake during night (give time & reason)? _____   _____

Did you wake up refreshed today or tired? ☐ Refreshed ☐ Tired   _____

Did you start slow this morning? ☐ Yes ☐ No   If yes, how long did it take to feel alert? _____

MOVEMENT :

Details: _____

_____

_____

GENERAL:

How did you feel today? _____

_____

OTHER INFO: _____

DAILY FOOD & LIFESTYLE DIARY

DAILY FOOD DIARY - DATE: _____

Complete everyday for 12 weeks

MEAL 1 – TIME: _____

Please fill out form 1-2 hours after each meal

Most likely too many carbs	Balanced Responses	Most likely too much protein &/or fat	
☐ Headache	☐ Appetite feels satisfied	☐ Lethargic	Approx. of macro Nutrient ratios of meal
☐ Anxiety	☐ Feel emotionally balanced	☐ Mentally Sluggish	% Carbs _____
☐ Jittery/wired	☐ Good mental focus	☐ Heavy Gut	% Protein _____
☐ Difficulty concentrating	☐ Normal level of energy	☐ Feel full yet still hungry	% Fat _____
☐ Hunger is not satisfied	☐ No cravings for sweets	☐ Crave sweets	Foods Eaten: _____
☐ Crave sweet	☐ No cravings for more food	☐ Crave Caffeine	_____
☐ Crave Protein & fat		(if more than hour after meal could	_____
		be a crash from too much carb)	_____

MEAL 2 – TIME: _____

Most likely too many carbs	Balanced Responses	Most likely too much protein &/or fat	
☐ Headache	☐ Appetite feels satisfied	☐ Lethargic	Approx. of macro Nutrient ratios of meal
☐ Anxiety	☐ Feel emotionally balanced	☐ Mentally Sluggish	% Carbs _____
☐ Jittery/wired	☐ Good mental focus	☐ Heavy Gut	% Protein _____
☐ Difficulty concentrating	☐ Normal level of energy	☐ Feel full yet still hungry	% Fat _____
☐ Hunger is not satisfied	☐ No cravings for sweets	☐ Crave sweets	Foods Eaten: _____
☐ Crave sweet	☐ No cravings for more food	☐ Crave Caffeine	_____
☐ Crave Protein & fat		(if more than hour after meal could	_____
		be a crash from too much carb)	_____

MEAL 3 – TIME: _____

Most likely too many carbs	Balanced Responses	Most likely too much protein &/or fat	
☐ Headache	☐ Appetite feels satisfied	☐ Lethargic	Approx. of macro Nutrient ratios of meal
☐ Anxiety	☐ Feel emotionally balanced	☐ Mentally Sluggish	% Carbs _____
☐ Jittery/wired	☐ Good mental focus	☐ Heavy Gut	% Protein _____
☐ Difficulty concentrating	☐ Normal level of energy	☐ Feel full yet still hungry	% Fat _____
☐ Hunger is not satisfied	☐ No cravings for sweets	☐ Crave sweets	Foods Eaten: _____
☐ Crave sweet	☐ No cravings for more food	☐ Crave Caffeine	_____
☐ Crave Protein & fat		(if more than hour after meal could	_____
		be a crash from too much carb)	_____

SNACKS:

Time: _____ Details: _____
Time: _____ Details: _____
Time: _____ Details: _____

DRINKS:

Details: _____
_____
_____

LIFESTYLE:

What time did you go to sleep?_____ What time did you get up? _____ Bowel movement(s)?
Sleep quality? ☐ Sound ☐ Restless Did you have night Sweats? ☐ Yes ☐ No (number, colour, size & shape)
Did you awake during night (give time & reason)? _____ _____
Did you wake up refreshed today or tired? ☐ Refreshed ☐ Tired _____
Did you start slow this morning? ☐ Yes ☐ No If yes, how long did it take to feel alert? _____

MOVEMENT :

Details: _____
_____
_____

GENERAL:

How did you feel today? _____
_____
_____

OTHER INFO: _____

DAILY FOOD & LIFESTYLE DIARY

DAILY FOOD DIARY - DATE: _____

Complete everyday for 12 weeks

MEAL 1 – TIME: _____

Please fill out form 1-2 hours after each meal

Most likely too many carbs
- ☐ Headache
- ☐ Anxiety
- ☐ Jittery/wired
- ☐ Difficulty concentrating
- ☐ Hunger is not satisfied
- ☐ Crave sweet
- ☐ Crave Protein & fat

Balanced Responses
- ☐ Appetite feels satisfied
- ☐ Feel emotionally balanced
- ☐ Good mental focus
- ☐ Normal level of energy
- ☐ No cravings for sweets
- ☐ No cravings for more food

Most likely too much protein &/or fat
- ☐ Lethargic
- ☐ Mentally Sluggish
- ☐ Heavy Gut
- ☐ Feel full yet still hungry
- ☐ Crave sweets
- ☐ Crave Caffeine
(if more than hour after meal could be a crash from too much carb)

Approx. of macro Nutrient ratios of meal
% Carbs _____
% Protein _____
% Fat _____
Foods Eaten: _____
_____
_____
_____
_____
_____

MEAL 2 – TIME: _____

Most likely too many carbs
- ☐ Headache
- ☐ Anxiety
- ☐ Jittery/wired
- ☐ Difficulty concentrating
- ☐ Hunger is not satisfied
- ☐ Crave sweet
- ☐ Crave Protein & fat

Balanced Responses
- ☐ Appetite feels satisfied
- ☐ Feel emotionally balanced
- ☐ Good mental focus
- ☐ Normal level of energy
- ☐ No cravings for sweets
- ☐ No cravings for more food

Most likely too much protein &/or fat
- ☐ Lethargic
- ☐ Mentally Sluggish
- ☐ Heavy Gut
- ☐ Feel full yet still hungry
- ☐ Crave sweets
- ☐ Crave Caffeine
(if more than hour after meal could be a crash from too much carb)

Approx. of macro Nutrient ratios of meal
% Carbs _____
% Protein _____
% Fat _____
Foods Eaten: _____
_____
_____
_____
_____
_____

MEAL 3 – TIME: _____

Most likely too many carbs
- ☐ Headache
- ☐ Anxiety
- ☐ Jittery/wired
- ☐ Difficulty concentrating
- ☐ Hunger is not satisfied
- ☐ Crave sweet
- ☐ Crave Protein & fat

Balanced Responses
- ☐ Appetite feels satisfied
- ☐ Feel emotionally balanced
- ☐ Good mental focus
- ☐ Normal level of energy
- ☐ No cravings for sweets
- ☐ No cravings for more food

Most likely too much protein &/or fat
- ☐ Lethargic
- ☐ Mentally Sluggish
- ☐ Heavy Gut
- ☐ Feel full yet still hungry
- ☐ Crave sweets
- ☐ Crave Caffeine
(if more than hour after meal could be a crash from too much carb)

Approx. of macro Nutrient ratios of meal
% Carbs _____
% Protein _____
% Fat _____
Foods Eaten: _____
_____
_____
_____
_____
_____

SNACKS:
Time: _____ Details: _____
Time: _____ Details: _____
Time: _____ Details: _____

DRINKS:
Details: _____
_____
_____

LIFESTYLE:
What time did you go to sleep?_____ What time did you get up? _____
Sleep quality? ☐ Sound ☐ Restless   Did you have night Sweats? ☐ Yes ☐ No
Did you awake during night (give time & reason)? _____
Did you wake up refreshed today or tired? ☐ Refreshed ☐ Tired
Did you start slow this morning? ☐ Yes ☐ No   If yes, how long did it take to feel alert? _____

Bowel movement(s)?
(number, colour, size & shape)
_____
_____

MOVEMENT :
Details: _____
_____
_____

GENERAL:
How did you feel today? _____
_____

OTHER INFO: _____

DAILY FOOD & LIFESTYLE DIARY

DAILY FOOD DIARY - DATE: _____

Complete everyday for 12 weeks

Please fill out form 1-2 hours after each meal

MEAL 1 – TIME: _____

Most likely too many carbs

- ☐ Headache
- ☐ Anxiety
- ☐ Jittery/wired
- ☐ Difficulty concentrating
- ☐ Hunger is not satisfied
- ☐ Crave sweet
- ☐ Crave Protein & fat

Balanced Responses

- ☐ Appetite feels satisfied
- ☐ Feel emotionally balanced
- ☐ Good mental focus
- ☐ Normal level of energy
- ☐ No cravings for sweets
- ☐ No cravings for more food

Most likely too much protein &/or fat

- ☐ Lethargic
- ☐ Mentally Sluggish
- ☐ Heavy Gut
- ☐ Feel full yet still hungry
- ☐ Crave sweets
- ☐ Crave Caffeine

(if more than hour after meal could be a crash from too much carb)

Approx. of macro Nutrient ratios of meal

% Carbs _____
% Protein _____
% Fat _____
Foods Eaten: _____
_____
_____
_____
_____
_____

MEAL 2 – TIME: _____

Most likely too many carbs

- ☐ Headache
- ☐ Anxiety
- ☐ Jittery/wired
- ☐ Difficulty concentrating
- ☐ Hunger is not satisfied
- ☐ Crave sweet
- ☐ Crave Protein & fat

Balanced Responses

- ☐ Appetite feels satisfied
- ☐ Feel emotionally balanced
- ☐ Good mental focus
- ☐ Normal level of energy
- ☐ No cravings for sweets
- ☐ No cravings for more food

Most likely too much protein &/or fat

- ☐ Lethargic
- ☐ Mentally Sluggish
- ☐ Heavy Gut
- ☐ Feel full yet still hungry
- ☐ Crave sweets
- ☐ Crave Caffeine

(if more than hour after meal could be a crash from too much carb)

Approx. of macro Nutrient ratios of meal

% Carbs _____
% Protein _____
% Fat _____
Foods Eaten: _____
_____
_____
_____
_____
_____

MEAL 3 – TIME: _____

Most likely too many carbs

- ☐ Headache
- ☐ Anxiety
- ☐ Jittery/wired
- ☐ Difficulty concentrating
- ☐ Hunger is not satisfied
- ☐ Crave sweet
- ☐ Crave Protein & fat

Balanced Responses

- ☐ Appetite feels satisfied
- ☐ Feel emotionally balanced
- ☐ Good mental focus
- ☐ Normal level of energy
- ☐ No cravings for sweets
- ☐ No cravings for more food

Most likely too much protein &/or fat

- ☐ Lethargic
- ☐ Mentally Sluggish
- ☐ Heavy Gut
- ☐ Feel full yet still hungry
- ☐ Crave sweets
- ☐ Crave Caffeine

(if more than hour after meal could be a crash from too much carb)

Approx. of macro Nutrient ratios of meal

% Carbs _____
% Protein _____
% Fat _____
Foods Eaten: _____
_____
_____
_____
_____
_____

SNACKS:

Time: _____ Details: _____
Time: _____ Details: _____
Time: _____ Details: _____

DRINKS:

Details: _____
_____
_____

LIFESTYLE:

What time did you go to sleep? _____ What time did you get up? _____
Sleep quality? ☐ Sound ☐ Restless   Did you have night Sweats? ☐ Yes ☐ No
Did you awake during night (give time & reason)? _____
Did you wake up refreshed today or tired? ☐ Refreshed ☐ Tired
Did you start slow this morning? ☐ Yes ☐ No   If yes, how long did it take to feel alert? _____

Bowel movement(s)?
(number, colour, size & shape)

_____
_____

MOVEMENT :

Details: _____
_____
_____

GENERAL:

How did you feel today? _____
_____
_____

OTHER INFO: _____

DAILY FOOD & LIFESTYLE DIARY

DAILY FOOD DIARY - DATE: _____

Complete everyday for 12 weeks

MEAL 1 – TIME: _____

Please fill out form 1-2 hours after each meal

Most likely too many carbs	Balanced Responses	Most likely too much protein &/or fat	Approx. of macro Nutrient ratios of meal

☐ Headache
☐ Anxiety
☐ Jittery/wired
☐ Difficulty concentrating
☐ Hunger is not satisfied
☐ Crave sweet
☐ Crave Protein & fat

Balanced Responses
☐ Appetite feels satisfied
☐ Feel emotionally balanced
☐ Good mental focus
☐ Normal level of energy
☐ No cravings for sweets
☐ No cravings for more food

Most likely too much protein &/or fat
☐ Lethargic
☐ Mentally Sluggish
☐ Heavy Gut
☐ Feel full yet still hungry
☐ Crave sweets
☐ Crave Caffeine
(if more than hour after meal could be a crash from too much carb)

Approx. of macro Nutrient ratios of meal
% Carbs _____
% Protein _____
% Fat _____
Foods Eaten: _____
_____
_____
_____
_____
_____

MEAL 2 – TIME: _____

Most likely too many carbs
☐ Headache
☐ Anxiety
☐ Jittery/wired
☐ Difficulty concentrating
☐ Hunger is not satisfied
☐ Crave sweet
☐ Crave Protein & fat

Balanced Responses
☐ Appetite feels satisfied
☐ Feel emotionally balanced
☐ Good mental focus
☐ Normal level of energy
☐ No cravings for sweets
☐ No cravings for more food

Most likely too much protein &/or fat
☐ Lethargic
☐ Mentally Sluggish
☐ Heavy Gut
☐ Feel full yet still hungry
☐ Crave sweets
☐ Crave Caffeine
(if more than hour after meal could be a crash from too much carb)

Approx. of macro Nutrient ratios of meal
% Carbs _____
% Protein _____
% Fat _____
Foods Eaten: _____
_____
_____
_____
_____
_____

MEAL 3 – TIME: _____

Most likely too many carbs
☐ Headache
☐ Anxiety
☐ Jittery/wired
☐ Difficulty concentrating
☐ Hunger is not satisfied
☐ Crave sweet
☐ Crave Protein & fat

Balanced Responses
☐ Appetite feels satisfied
☐ Feel emotionally balanced
☐ Good mental focus
☐ Normal level of energy
☐ No cravings for sweets
☐ No cravings for more food

Most likely too much protein &/or fat
☐ Lethargic
☐ Mentally Sluggish
☐ Heavy Gut
☐ Feel full yet still hungry
☐ Crave sweets
☐ Crave Caffeine
(if more than hour after meal could be a crash from too much carb)

Approx. of macro Nutrient ratios of meal
% Carbs _____
% Protein _____
% Fat _____
Foods Eaten: _____
_____
_____
_____
_____

SNACKS:

Time: _____ Details: _____
Time: _____ Details: _____
Time: _____ Details: _____

DRINKS:

Details: _____
_____
_____

LIFESTYLE:

What time did you go to sleep? _____ What time did you get up? _____
Sleep quality? ☐ Sound ☐ Restless   Did you have night Sweats? ☐ Yes ☐ No
Did you awake during night (give time & reason)? _____
Did you wake up refreshed today or tired? ☐ Refreshed ☐ Tired
Did you start slow this morning? ☐ Yes ☐ No   If yes, how long did it take to feel alert? _____

Bowel movement(s)?
(number, colour, size & shape)
_____
_____

MOVEMENT :

Details: _____
_____
_____

GENERAL:

How did you feel today? _____
_____
_____

OTHER INFO: _____

DAILY FOOD & LIFESTYLE DIARY

DAILY FOOD DIARY - DATE: _____

Complete everyday for 12 weeks

MEAL 1 – TIME: _____

Please fill out form 1-2 hours after each meal

Most likely too many carbs	Balanced Responses	Most likely too much protein &/or fat	
☐ Headache	☐ Appetite feels satisfied	☐ Lethargic	Approx. of macro Nutrient ratios of meal
☐ Anxiety	☐ Feel emotionally balanced	☐ Mentally Sluggish	% Carbs _____
☐ Jittery/wired	☐ Good mental focus	☐ Heavy Gut	% Protein _____
☐ Difficulty concentrating	☐ Normal level of energy	☐ Feel full yet still hungry	% Fat _____
☐ Hunger is not satisfied	☐ No cravings for sweets	☐ Crave sweets	Foods Eaten: _____
☐ Crave sweet	☐ No cravings for more food	☐ Crave Caffeine	_____
☐ Crave Protein & fat		(if more than hour after meal could be a crash from too much carb)	_____

MEAL 2 – TIME: _____

Most likely too many carbs	Balanced Responses	Most likely too much protein &/or fat	
☐ Headache	☐ Appetite feels satisfied	☐ Lethargic	Approx. of macro Nutrient ratios of meal
☐ Anxiety	☐ Feel emotionally balanced	☐ Mentally Sluggish	% Carbs _____
☐ Jittery/wired	☐ Good mental focus	☐ Heavy Gut	% Protein _____
☐ Difficulty concentrating	☐ Normal level of energy	☐ Feel full yet still hungry	% Fat _____
☐ Hunger is not satisfied	☐ No cravings for sweets	☐ Crave sweets	Foods Eaten: _____
☐ Crave sweet	☐ No cravings for more food	☐ Crave Caffeine	_____
☐ Crave Protein & fat		(if more than hour after meal could be a crash from too much carb)	_____

MEAL 3 – TIME: _____

Most likely too many carbs	Balanced Responses	Most likely too much protein &/or fat	
☐ Headache	☐ Appetite feels satisfied	☐ Lethargic	Approx. of macro Nutrient ratios of meal
☐ Anxiety	☐ Feel emotionally balanced	☐ Mentally Sluggish	% Carbs _____
☐ Jittery/wired	☐ Good mental focus	☐ Heavy Gut	% Protein _____
☐ Difficulty concentrating	☐ Normal level of energy	☐ Feel full yet still hungry	% Fat _____
☐ Hunger is not satisfied	☐ No cravings for sweets	☐ Crave sweets	Foods Eaten: _____
☐ Crave sweet	☐ No cravings for more food	☐ Crave Caffeine	_____
☐ Crave Protein & fat		(if more than hour after meal could be a crash from too much carb)	_____

SNACKS:

Time: _____ Details: _____
Time: _____ Details: _____
Time: _____ Details: _____

DRINKS:

Details: _____
_____
_____

LIFESTYLE:

What time did you go to sleep? _____ What time did you get up? _____ Bowel movement(s)?
Sleep quality? ☐ Sound ☐ Restless   Did you have night Sweats? ☐ Yes ☐ No   (number, colour, size & shape)
Did you awake during night (give time & reason)? _____   _____
Did you wake up refreshed today or tired? ☐ Refreshed ☐ Tired   _____
Did you start slow this morning? ☐ Yes ☐ No   If yes, how long did it take to feel alert? _____

MOVEMENT :

Details: _____
_____
_____

GENERAL:

How did you feel today? _____
_____

OTHER INFO: _____

DAILY FOOD & LIFESTYLE DIARY

DAILY FOOD DIARY - DATE: _____

Complete everyday for 12 weeks

MEAL 1 – TIME: _____

Please fill out form 1-2 hours after each meal

Most likely too many carbs

- ☐ Headache
- ☐ Anxiety
- ☐ Jittery/wired
- ☐ Difficulty concentrating
- ☐ Hunger is not satisfied
- ☐ Crave sweet
- ☐ Crave Protein & fat

Balanced Responses

- ☐ Appetite feels satisfied
- ☐ Feel emotionally balanced
- ☐ Good mental focus
- ☐ Normal level of energy
- ☐ No cravings for sweets
- ☐ No cravings for more food

Most likely too much protein &/or fat

- ☐ Lethargic
- ☐ Mentally Sluggish
- ☐ Heavy Gut
- ☐ Feel full yet still hungry
- ☐ Crave sweets
- ☐ Crave Caffeine

(if more than hour after meal could be a crash from too much carb)

Approx. of macro Nutrient ratios of meal
% Carbs _____
% Protein _____
% Fat _____
Foods Eaten: _____
_____
_____
_____
_____
_____

MEAL 2 – TIME: _____

Most likely too many carbs

- ☐ Headache
- ☐ Anxiety
- ☐ Jittery/wired
- ☐ Difficulty concentrating
- ☐ Hunger is not satisfied
- ☐ Crave sweet
- ☐ Crave Protein & fat

Balanced Responses

- ☐ Appetite feels satisfied
- ☐ Feel emotionally balanced
- ☐ Good mental focus
- ☐ Normal level of energy
- ☐ No cravings for sweets
- ☐ No cravings for more food

Most likely too much protein &/or fat

- ☐ Lethargic
- ☐ Mentally Sluggish
- ☐ Heavy Gut
- ☐ Feel full yet still hungry
- ☐ Crave sweets
- ☐ Crave Caffeine

(if more than hour after meal could be a crash from too much carb)

Approx. of macro Nutrient ratios of meal
% Carbs _____
% Protein _____
% Fat _____
Foods Eaten: _____
_____
_____
_____
_____
_____

MEAL 3 – TIME: _____

Most likely too many carbs

- ☐ Headache
- ☐ Anxiety
- ☐ Jittery/wired
- ☐ Difficulty concentrating
- ☐ Hunger is not satisfied
- ☐ Crave sweet
- ☐ Crave Protein & fat

Balanced Responses

- ☐ Appetite feels satisfied
- ☐ Feel emotionally balanced
- ☐ Good mental focus
- ☐ Normal level of energy
- ☐ No cravings for sweets
- ☐ No cravings for more food

Most likely too much protein &/or fat

- ☐ Lethargic
- ☐ Mentally Sluggish
- ☐ Heavy Gut
- ☐ Feel full yet still hungry
- ☐ Crave sweets
- ☐ Crave Caffeine

(if more than hour after meal could be a crash from too much carb)

Approx. of macro Nutrient ratios of meal
% Carbs _____
% Protein _____
% Fat _____
Foods Eaten: _____
_____
_____
_____
_____
_____

SNACKS:

Time: _____ Details: _____
Time: _____ Details: _____
Time: _____ Details: _____

DRINKS:

Details: _____
_____
_____

LIFESTYLE:

What time did you go to sleep?_____ What time did you get up? _____
Sleep quality? ☐ Sound ☐ Restless   Did you have night Sweats? ☐ Yes ☐ No
Did you awake during night (give time & reason)? _____
Did you wake up refreshed today or tired? ☐ Refreshed ☐ Tired
Did you start slow this morning? ☐ Yes ☐ No   If yes, how long did it take to feel alert? _____

Bowel movement(s)?
(number, colour, size & shape)
_____
_____

MOVEMENT :

Details:_____
_____
_____

GENERAL:

How did you feel today? _____
_____

OTHER INFO: _____

DAILY FOOD & LIFESTYLE DIARY

DAILY FOOD DIARY - DATE: _____

Complete everyday for 12 weeks

MEAL 1 – TIME: _____

Please fill out form 1-2 hours after each meal

Most likely too many carbs

- ☐ Headache
- ☐ Anxiety
- ☐ Jittery/wired
- ☐ Difficulty concentrating
- ☐ Hunger is not satisfied
- ☐ Crave sweet
- ☐ Crave Protein & fat

Balanced Responses

- ☐ Appetite feels satisfied
- ☐ Feel emotionally balanced
- ☐ Good mental focus
- ☐ Normal level of energy
- ☐ No cravings for sweets
- ☐ No cravings for more food

Most likely too much protein &/or fat

- ☐ Lethargic
- ☐ Mentally Sluggish
- ☐ Heavy Gut
- ☐ Feel full yet still hungry
- ☐ Crave sweets
- ☐ Crave Caffeine

(if more than hour after meal could be a crash from too much carb)

Approx. of macro Nutrient ratios of meal
% Carbs _____
% Protein _____
% Fat _____
Foods Eaten: _____
_____
_____
_____
_____

MEAL 2 – TIME: _____

Most likely too many carbs

- ☐ Headache
- ☐ Anxiety
- ☐ Jittery/wired
- ☐ Difficulty concentrating
- ☐ Hunger is not satisfied
- ☐ Crave sweet
- ☐ Crave Protein & fat

Balanced Responses

- ☐ Appetite feels satisfied
- ☐ Feel emotionally balanced
- ☐ Good mental focus
- ☐ Normal level of energy
- ☐ No cravings for sweets
- ☐ No cravings for more food

Most likely too much protein &/or fat

- ☐ Lethargic
- ☐ Mentally Sluggish
- ☐ Heavy Gut
- ☐ Feel full yet still hungry
- ☐ Crave sweets
- ☐ Crave Caffeine

(if more than hour after meal could be a crash from too much carb)

Approx. of macro Nutrient ratios of meal
% Carbs _____
% Protein _____
% Fat _____
Foods Eaten: _____
_____
_____
_____
_____

MEAL 3 – TIME: _____

Most likely too many carbs

- ☐ Headache
- ☐ Anxiety
- ☐ Jittery/wired
- ☐ Difficulty concentrating
- ☐ Hunger is not satisfied
- ☐ Crave sweet
- ☐ Crave Protein & fat

Balanced Responses

- ☐ Appetite feels satisfied
- ☐ Feel emotionally balanced
- ☐ Good mental focus
- ☐ Normal level of energy
- ☐ No cravings for sweets
- ☐ No cravings for more food

Most likely too much protein &/or fat

- ☐ Lethargic
- ☐ Mentally Sluggish
- ☐ Heavy Gut
- ☐ Feel full yet still hungry
- ☐ Crave sweets
- ☐ Crave Caffeine

(if more than hour after meal could be a crash from too much carb)

Approx. of macro Nutrient ratios of meal
% Carbs _____
% Protein _____
% Fat _____
Foods Eaten: _____
_____
_____
_____
_____

SNACKS:

Time: _____ Details: _____
Time: _____ Details: _____
Time: _____ Details: _____

DRINKS:

Details: _____
_____
_____

LIFESTYLE:

What time did you go to sleep?_____ What time did you get up? _____
Sleep quality? ☐ Sound ☐ Restless   Did you have night Sweats? ☐ Yes ☐ No
Did you awake during night (give time & reason)? _____
Did you wake up refreshed today or tired? ☐ Refreshed ☐ Tired
Did you start slow this morning? ☐ Yes ☐ No   If yes, how long did it take to feel alert? _____

Bowel movement(s)?
(number, colour, size & shape)
_____
_____

MOVEMENT :

Details:_____
_____
_____

GENERAL:

How did you feel today? _____
_____
_____

OTHER INFO: _____

DAILY FOOD & LIFESTYLE DIARY

DAILY FOOD DIARY - DATE: _____

MEAL 1 – TIME: _____

Complete everyday for 12 weeks

Please fill out form 1-2 hours after each meal

Most likely too many carbs
- ☐ Headache
- ☐ Anxiety
- ☐ Jittery/wired
- ☐ Difficulty concentrating
- ☐ Hunger is not satisfied
- ☐ Crave sweet
- ☐ Crave Protein & fat

Balanced Responses
- ☐ Appetite feels satisfied
- ☐ Feel emotionally balanced
- ☐ Good mental focus
- ☐ Normal level of energy
- ☐ No cravings for sweets
- ☐ No cravings for more food

Most likely too much protein &/or fat
- ☐ Lethargic
- ☐ Mentally Sluggish
- ☐ Heavy Gut
- ☐ Feel full yet still hungry
- ☐ Crave sweets
- ☐ Crave Caffeine

(if more than hour after meal could be a crash from too much carb)

Approx. of macro Nutrient ratios of meal
% Carbs _____
% Protein _____
% Fat _____
Foods Eaten: _____
_____
_____
_____
_____

MEAL 2 – TIME: _____

Most likely too many carbs
- ☐ Headache
- ☐ Anxiety
- ☐ Jittery/wired
- ☐ Difficulty concentrating
- ☐ Hunger is not satisfied
- ☐ Crave sweet
- ☐ Crave Protein & fat

Balanced Responses
- ☐ Appetite feels satisfied
- ☐ Feel emotionally balanced
- ☐ Good mental focus
- ☐ Normal level of energy
- ☐ No cravings for sweets
- ☐ No cravings for more food

Most likely too much protein &/or fat
- ☐ Lethargic
- ☐ Mentally Sluggish
- ☐ Heavy Gut
- ☐ Feel full yet still hungry
- ☐ Crave sweets
- ☐ Crave Caffeine

(if more than hour after meal could be a crash from too much carb)

Approx. of macro Nutrient ratios of meal
% Carbs _____
% Protein _____
% Fat _____
Foods Eaten: _____
_____
_____
_____
_____

MEAL 3 – TIME: _____

Most likely too many carbs
- ☐ Headache
- ☐ Anxiety
- ☐ Jittery/wired
- ☐ Difficulty concentrating
- ☐ Hunger is not satisfied
- ☐ Crave sweet
- ☐ Crave Protein & fat

Balanced Responses
- ☐ Appetite feels satisfied
- ☐ Feel emotionally balanced
- ☐ Good mental focus
- ☐ Normal level of energy
- ☐ No cravings for sweets
- ☐ No cravings for more food

Most likely too much protein &/or fat
- ☐ Lethargic
- ☐ Mentally Sluggish
- ☐ Heavy Gut
- ☐ Feel full yet still hungry
- ☐ Crave sweets
- ☐ Crave Caffeine

(if more than hour after meal could be a crash from too much carb)

Approx. of macro Nutrient ratios of meal
% Carbs _____
% Protein _____
% Fat _____
Foods Eaten: _____
_____
_____
_____
_____

SNACKS:

Time: _____ Details: _____
Time: _____ Details: _____
Time: _____ Details: _____

DRINKS:

Details: _____
_____
_____

LIFESTYLE:

What time did you go to sleep?_____ What time did you get up? _____

Sleep quality? ☐ Sound ☐ Restless   Did you have night Sweats? ☐ Yes ☐ No

Did you awake during night (give time & reason)? _____

Did you wake up refreshed today or tired? ☐ Refreshed ☐ Tired

Did you start slow this morning? ☐ Yes ☐ No   If yes, how long did it take to feel alert? _____

Bowel movement(s)?
(number, colour, size & shape)
_____
_____

MOVEMENT :

Details:_____
_____
_____

GENERAL:

How did you feel today? _____
_____
_____

OTHER INFO: _____

DAILY FOOD & LIFESTYLE DIARY

DAILY FOOD DIARY - DATE: _____

MEAL 1 – TIME: _____

Complete everyday for 12 weeks

Please fill out form 1-2 hours after each meal

Most likely too many carbs	Balanced Responses	Most likely too much protein &/or fat	
☐ Headache	☐ Appetite feels satisfied	☐ Lethargic	Approx. of macro Nutrient ratios of meal
☐ Anxiety	☐ Feel emotionally balanced	☐ Mentally Sluggish	% Carbs _____
☐ Jittery/wired	☐ Good mental focus	☐ Heavy Gut	% Protein _____
☐ Difficulty concentrating	☐ Normal level of energy	☐ Feel full yet still hungry	% Fat _____
☐ Hunger is not satisfied	☐ No cravings for sweets	☐ Crave sweets	Foods Eaten: _____
☐ Crave sweet	☐ No cravings for more food	☐ Crave Caffeine	_____
☐ Crave Protein & fat		(if more than hour after meal could	_____
		be a crash from too much carb)	_____

MEAL 2 – TIME: _____

Most likely too many carbs	Balanced Responses	Most likely too much protein &/or fat	
☐ Headache	☐ Appetite feels satisfied	☐ Lethargic	Approx. of macro Nutrient ratios of meal
☐ Anxiety	☐ Feel emotionally balanced	☐ Mentally Sluggish	% Carbs _____
☐ Jittery/wired	☐ Good mental focus	☐ Heavy Gut	% Protein _____
☐ Difficulty concentrating	☐ Normal level of energy	☐ Feel full yet still hungry	% Fat _____
☐ Hunger is not satisfied	☐ No cravings for sweets	☐ Crave sweets	Foods Eaten: _____
☐ Crave sweet	☐ No cravings for more food	☐ Crave Caffeine	_____
☐ Crave Protein & fat		(if more than hour after meal could	_____
		be a crash from too much carb)	_____

MEAL 3 – TIME: _____

Most likely too many carbs	Balanced Responses	Most likely too much protein &/or fat	
☐ Headache	☐ Appetite feels satisfied	☐ Lethargic	Approx. of macro Nutrient ratios of meal
☐ Anxiety	☐ Feel emotionally balanced	☐ Mentally Sluggish	% Carbs _____
☐ Jittery/wired	☐ Good mental focus	☐ Heavy Gut	% Protein _____
☐ Difficulty concentrating	☐ Normal level of energy	☐ Feel full yet still hungry	% Fat _____
☐ Hunger is not satisfied	☐ No cravings for sweets	☐ Crave sweets	Foods Eaten: _____
☐ Crave sweet	☐ No cravings for more food	☐ Crave Caffeine	_____
☐ Crave Protein & fat		(if more than hour after meal could	_____
		be a crash from too much carb)	_____

SNACKS:

Time: _____ Details: _____

Time: _____ Details: _____

Time: _____ Details: _____

DRINKS:

Details: _____

_____

_____

LIFESTYLE:

What time did you go to sleep? _____ What time did you get up? _____

Sleep quality? ☐ Sound ☐ Restless   Did you have night Sweats? ☐ Yes ☐ No

Did you awake during night (give time & reason)? _____

Did you wake up refreshed today or tired? ☐ Refreshed ☐ Tired

Did you start slow this morning? ☐ Yes ☐ No   If yes, how long did it take to feel alert? _____

Bowel movement(s)?
(number, colour, size & shape)

_____

_____

MOVEMENT :

Details: _____

_____

_____

GENERAL:

How did you feel today? _____

_____

_____

OTHER INFO: _____

DAILY FOOD & LIFESTYLE DIARY

DAILY FOOD DIARY - DATE: _____

Complete everyday for 12 weeks

Please fill out form 1-2 hours after each meal

MEAL 1 – TIME: _____

Most likely too many carbs	Balanced Responses	Most likely too much protein &/or fat	Approx. of macro Nutrient ratios of meal

Most likely too many carbs
- ☐ Headache
- ☐ Anxiety
- ☐ Jittery/wired
- ☐ Difficulty concentrating
- ☐ Hunger is not satisfied
- ☐ Crave sweet
- ☐ Crave Protein & fat

Balanced Responses
- ☐ Appetite feels satisfied
- ☐ Feel emotionally balanced
- ☐ Good mental focus
- ☐ Normal level of energy
- ☐ No cravings for sweets
- ☐ No cravings for more food

Most likely too much protein &/or fat
- ☐ Lethargic
- ☐ Mentally Sluggish
- ☐ Heavy Gut
- ☐ Feel full yet still hungry
- ☐ Crave sweets
- ☐ Crave Caffeine
(if more than hour after meal could be a crash from too much carb)

Approx. of macro Nutrient ratios of meal
% Carbs _____
% Protein _____
% Fat _____
Foods Eaten: _____
_____
_____
_____
_____
_____

MEAL 2 – TIME: _____

Most likely too many carbs
- ☐ Headache
- ☐ Anxiety
- ☐ Jittery/wired
- ☐ Difficulty concentrating
- ☐ Hunger is not satisfied
- ☐ Crave sweet
- ☐ Crave Protein & fat

Balanced Responses
- ☐ Appetite feels satisfied
- ☐ Feel emotionally balanced
- ☐ Good mental focus
- ☐ Normal level of energy
- ☐ No cravings for sweets
- ☐ No cravings for more food

Most likely too much protein &/or fat
- ☐ Lethargic
- ☐ Mentally Sluggish
- ☐ Heavy Gut
- ☐ Feel full yet still hungry
- ☐ Crave sweets
- ☐ Crave Caffeine
(if more than hour after meal could be a crash from too much carb)

Approx. of macro Nutrient ratios of meal
% Carbs _____
% Protein _____
% Fat _____
Foods Eaten: _____
_____
_____
_____
_____
_____

MEAL 3 – TIME: _____

Most likely too many carbs
- ☐ Headache
- ☐ Anxiety
- ☐ Jittery/wired
- ☐ Difficulty concentrating
- ☐ Hunger is not satisfied
- ☐ Crave sweet
- ☐ Crave Protein & fat

Balanced Responses
- ☐ Appetite feels satisfied
- ☐ Feel emotionally balanced
- ☐ Good mental focus
- ☐ Normal level of energy
- ☐ No cravings for sweets
- ☐ No cravings for more food

Most likely too much protein &/or fat
- ☐ Lethargic
- ☐ Mentally Sluggish
- ☐ Heavy Gut
- ☐ Feel full yet still hungry
- ☐ Crave sweets
- ☐ Crave Caffeine
(if more than hour after meal could be a crash from too much carb)

Approx. of macro Nutrient ratios of meal
% Carbs _____
% Protein _____
% Fat _____
Foods Eaten: _____
_____
_____
_____
_____
_____

SNACKS:
Time: _____ Details: _____
Time: _____ Details: _____
Time: _____ Details: _____

DRINKS:
Details: _____
_____
_____

LIFESTYLE:
What time did you go to sleep? _____ What time did you get up? _____

Sleep quality? ☐ Sound ☐ Restless   Did you have night Sweats? ☐ Yes ☐ No

Did you awake during night (give time & reason)? _____

Did you wake up refreshed today or tired? ☐ Refreshed ☐ Tired

Did you start slow this morning? ☐ Yes ☐ No   If yes, how long did it take to feel alert? _____

Bowel movement(s)?
(number, colour, size & shape)
_____
_____

MOVEMENT :
Details: _____
_____
_____

GENERAL:
How did you feel today? _____
_____
_____

OTHER INFO: _____

DAILY FOOD & LIFESTYLE DIARY

DAILY FOOD DIARY - DATE: _____

Complete everyday for 12 weeks

MEAL 1 – TIME: _____

Please fill out form 1-2 hours after each meal

Most likely too many carbs	Balanced Responses	Most likely too much protein &/or fat	
☐ Headache	☐ Appetite feels satisfied	☐ Lethargic	Approx. of macro Nutrient ratios of meal
☐ Anxiety	☐ Feel emotionally balanced	☐ Mentally Sluggish	% Carbs _____
☐ Jittery/wired	☐ Good mental focus	☐ Heavy Gut	% Protein _____
☐ Difficulty concentrating	☐ Normal level of energy	☐ Feel full yet still hungry	% Fat _____
☐ Hunger is not satisfied	☐ No cravings for sweets	☐ Crave sweets	Foods Eaten: _____
☐ Crave sweet	☐ No cravings for more food	☐ Crave Caffeine	_____
☐ Crave Protein & fat		(if more than hour after meal could be a crash from too much carb)	_____

MEAL 2 – TIME: _____

Most likely too many carbs	Balanced Responses	Most likely too much protein &/or fat	
☐ Headache	☐ Appetite feels satisfied	☐ Lethargic	Approx. of macro Nutrient ratios of meal
☐ Anxiety	☐ Feel emotionally balanced	☐ Mentally Sluggish	% Carbs _____
☐ Jittery/wired	☐ Good mental focus	☐ Heavy Gut	% Protein _____
☐ Difficulty concentrating	☐ Normal level of energy	☐ Feel full yet still hungry	% Fat _____
☐ Hunger is not satisfied	☐ No cravings for sweets	☐ Crave sweets	Foods Eaten: _____
☐ Crave sweet	☐ No cravings for more food	☐ Crave Caffeine	_____
☐ Crave Protein & fat		(if more than hour after meal could be a crash from too much carb)	_____

MEAL 3 – TIME: _____

Most likely too many carbs	Balanced Responses	Most likely too much protein &/or fat	
☐ Headache	☐ Appetite feels satisfied	☐ Lethargic	Approx. of macro Nutrient ratios of meal
☐ Anxiety	☐ Feel emotionally balanced	☐ Mentally Sluggish	% Carbs _____
☐ Jittery/wired	☐ Good mental focus	☐ Heavy Gut	% Protein _____
☐ Difficulty concentrating	☐ Normal level of energy	☐ Feel full yet still hungry	% Fat _____
☐ Hunger is not satisfied	☐ No cravings for sweets	☐ Crave sweets	Foods Eaten: _____
☐ Crave sweet	☐ No cravings for more food	☐ Crave Caffeine	_____
☐ Crave Protein & fat		(if more than hour after meal could be a crash from too much carb)	_____

SNACKS:

Time: _____ Details: _____

Time: _____ Details: _____

Time: _____ Details: _____

DRINKS:

Details: _____

_____

_____

LIFESTYLE:

What time did you go to sleep? _____ What time did you get up? _____

Sleep quality? ☐ Sound ☐ Restless   Did you have night Sweats? ☐ Yes ☐ No

Did you awake during night (give time & reason)? _____

Did you wake up refreshed today or tired? ☐ Refreshed ☐ Tired

Did you start slow this morning? ☐ Yes ☐ No   If yes, how long did it take to feel alert? _____

Bowel movement(s)?
(number, colour, size & shape)

_____

_____

MOVEMENT :

Details: _____

_____

_____

GENERAL:

How did you feel today? _____

_____

_____

OTHER INFO: _____

DAILY FOOD & LIFESTYLE DIARY

DAILY FOOD DIARY - DATE: _____

Complete everyday for 12 weeks

MEAL 1 – TIME: _____

Please fill out form 1-2 hours after each meal

Most likely too many carbs

☐ Headache
☐ Anxiety
☐ Jittery/wired
☐ Difficulty concentrating
☐ Hunger is not satisfied
☐ Crave sweet
☐ Crave Protein & fat

Balanced Responses

☐ Appetite feels satisfied
☐ Feel emotionally balanced
☐ Good mental focus
☐ Normal level of energy
☐ No cravings for sweets
☐ No cravings for more food

Most likely too much protein &/or fat

☐ Lethargic
☐ Mentally Sluggish
☐ Heavy Gut
☐ Feel full yet still hungry
☐ Crave sweets
☐ Crave Caffeine
(if more than hour after meal could
be a crash from too much carb)

Approx. of macro Nutrient ratios of meal
% Carbs _____
% Protein _____
% Fat _____
Foods Eaten: _____
_____
_____
_____
_____
_____

MEAL 2 – TIME: _____

Most likely too many carbs

☐ Headache
☐ Anxiety
☐ Jittery/wired
☐ Difficulty concentrating
☐ Hunger is not satisfied
☐ Crave sweet
☐ Crave Protein & fat

Balanced Responses

☐ Appetite feels satisfied
☐ Feel emotionally balanced
☐ Good mental focus
☐ Normal level of energy
☐ No cravings for sweets
☐ No cravings for more food

Most likely too much protein &/or fat

☐ Lethargic
☐ Mentally Sluggish
☐ Heavy Gut
☐ Feel full yet still hungry
☐ Crave sweets
☐ Crave Caffeine
(if more than hour after meal could
be a crash from too much carb)

Approx. of macro Nutrient ratios of meal
% Carbs _____
% Protein _____
% Fat _____
Foods Eaten: _____
_____
_____
_____
_____
_____

MEAL 3 – TIME: _____

Most likely too many carbs

☐ Headache
☐ Anxiety
☐ Jittery/wired
☐ Difficulty concentrating
☐ Hunger is not satisfied
☐ Crave sweet
☐ Crave Protein & fat

Balanced Responses

☐ Appetite feels satisfied
☐ Feel emotionally balanced
☐ Good mental focus
☐ Normal level of energy
☐ No cravings for sweets
☐ No cravings for more food

Most likely too much protein &/or fat

☐ Lethargic
☐ Mentally Sluggish
☐ Heavy Gut
☐ Feel full yet still hungry
☐ Crave sweets
☐ Crave Caffeine
(if more than hour after meal could
be a crash from too much carb)

Approx. of macro Nutrient ratios of meal
% Carbs _____
% Protein _____
% Fat _____
Foods Eaten: _____
_____
_____
_____
_____
_____

SNACKS:

Time: _____ Details: _____
Time: _____ Details: _____
Time: _____ Details: _____

DRINKS:

Details: _____
_____
_____

LIFESTYLE:

What time did you go to sleep?_____ What time did you get up? _____
Sleep quality? ☐ Sound ☐ Restless Did you have night Sweats? ☐ Yes ☐ No
Did you awake during night (give time & reason)? _____
Did you wake up refreshed today or tired? ☐ Refreshed ☐ Tired
Did you start slow this morning? ☐ Yes ☐ No If yes, how long did it take to feel alert? _____

Bowel movement(s)?
(number, colour, size & shape)
_____
_____

MOVEMENT :

Details:_____
_____
_____

GENERAL:

How did you feel today? _____
_____
_____

OTHER INFO: _____

DAILY FOOD & LIFESTYLE DIARY

DAILY FOOD DIARY - DATE: _____

Complete everyday for 12 weeks

MEAL 1 – TIME: _____

Please fill out form 1-2 hours after each meal

Most likely too many carbs

- [ ] Headache
- [ ] Anxiety
- [ ] Jittery/wired
- [ ] Difficulty concentrating
- [ ] Hunger is not satisfied
- [ ] Crave sweet
- [ ] Crave Protein & fat

Balanced Responses

- [ ] Appetite feels satisfied
- [ ] Feel emotionally balanced
- [ ] Good mental focus
- [ ] Normal level of energy
- [ ] No cravings for sweets
- [ ] No cravings for more food

Most likely too much protein &/or fat

- [ ] Lethargic
- [ ] Mentally Sluggish
- [ ] Heavy Gut
- [ ] Feel full yet still hungry
- [ ] Crave sweets
- [ ] Crave Caffeine

(if more than hour after meal could be a crash from too much carb)

Approx. of macro Nutrient ratios of meal

% Carbs _____
% Protein _____
% Fat _____
Foods Eaten: _____
_____
_____
_____
_____
_____

MEAL 2 – TIME: _____

Most likely too many carbs

- [ ] Headache
- [ ] Anxiety
- [ ] Jittery/wired
- [ ] Difficulty concentrating
- [ ] Hunger is not satisfied
- [ ] Crave sweet
- [ ] Crave Protein & fat

Balanced Responses

- [ ] Appetite feels satisfied
- [ ] Feel emotionally balanced
- [ ] Good mental focus
- [ ] Normal level of energy
- [ ] No cravings for sweets
- [ ] No cravings for more food

Most likely too much protein &/or fat

- [ ] Lethargic
- [ ] Mentally Sluggish
- [ ] Heavy Gut
- [ ] Feel full yet still hungry
- [ ] Crave sweets
- [ ] Crave Caffeine

(if more than hour after meal could be a crash from too much carb)

Approx. of macro Nutrient ratios of meal

% Carbs _____
% Protein _____
% Fat _____
Foods Eaten: _____
_____
_____
_____
_____
_____

MEAL 3 – TIME: _____

Most likely too many carbs

- [ ] Headache
- [ ] Anxiety
- [ ] Jittery/wired
- [ ] Difficulty concentrating
- [ ] Hunger is not satisfied
- [ ] Crave sweet
- [ ] Crave Protein & fat

Balanced Responses

- [ ] Appetite feels satisfied
- [ ] Feel emotionally balanced
- [ ] Good mental focus
- [ ] Normal level of energy
- [ ] No cravings for sweets
- [ ] No cravings for more food

Most likely too much protein &/or fat

- [ ] Lethargic
- [ ] Mentally Sluggish
- [ ] Heavy Gut
- [ ] Feel full yet still hungry
- [ ] Crave sweets
- [ ] Crave Caffeine

(if more than hour after meal could be a crash from too much carb)

Approx. of macro Nutrient ratios of meal

% Carbs _____
% Protein _____
% Fat _____
Foods Eaten: _____
_____
_____
_____
_____
_____

SNACKS:

Time: _____ Details: _____
Time: _____ Details: _____
Time: _____ Details: _____

DRINKS:

Details: _____
_____
_____

LIFESTYLE:

What time did you go to sleep? _____ What time did you get up? _____
Sleep quality? ☐ Sound ☐ Restless   Did you have night Sweats? ☐ Yes ☐ No
Did you awake during night (give time & reason)? _____
Did you wake up refreshed today or tired? ☐ Refreshed ☐ Tired
Did you start slow this morning? ☐ Yes ☐ No   If yes, how long did it take to feel alert? _____

Bowel movement(s)?
(number, colour, size & shape)
_____
_____

MOVEMENT :

Details: _____
_____
_____

GENERAL:

How did you feel today? _____
_____
_____

OTHER INFO: _____

DAILY FOOD & LIFESTYLE DIARY

DAILY FOOD DIARY - DATE: _____

Complete everyday for 12 weeks

Please fill out form 1-2 hours after each meal

MEAL 1 – TIME: _____

Most likely too many carbs
- ☐ Headache
- ☐ Anxiety
- ☐ Jittery/wired
- ☐ Difficulty concentrating
- ☐ Hunger is not satisfied
- ☐ Crave sweet
- ☐ Crave Protein & fat

Balanced Responses
- ☐ Appetite feels satisfied
- ☐ Feel emotionally balanced
- ☐ Good mental focus
- ☐ Normal level of energy
- ☐ No cravings for sweets
- ☐ No cravings for more food

Most likely too much protein &/or fat
- ☐ Lethargic
- ☐ Mentally Sluggish
- ☐ Heavy Gut
- ☐ Feel full yet still hungry
- ☐ Crave sweets
- ☐ Crave Caffeine
(if more than hour after meal could be a crash from too much carb)

Approx. of macro Nutrient ratios of meal
% Carbs _____
% Protein _____
% Fat _____
Foods Eaten: _____
_____
_____
_____
_____
_____

MEAL 2 – TIME: _____

Most likely too many carbs
- ☐ Headache
- ☐ Anxiety
- ☐ Jittery/wired
- ☐ Difficulty concentrating
- ☐ Hunger is not satisfied
- ☐ Crave sweet
- ☐ Crave Protein & fat

Balanced Responses
- ☐ Appetite feels satisfied
- ☐ Feel emotionally balanced
- ☐ Good mental focus
- ☐ Normal level of energy
- ☐ No cravings for sweets
- ☐ No cravings for more food

Most likely too much protein &/or fat
- ☐ Lethargic
- ☐ Mentally Sluggish
- ☐ Heavy Gut
- ☐ Feel full yet still hungry
- ☐ Crave sweets
- ☐ Crave Caffeine
(if more than hour after meal could be a crash from too much carb)

Approx. of macro Nutrient ratios of meal
% Carbs _____
% Protein _____
% Fat _____
Foods Eaten: _____
_____
_____
_____
_____
_____

MEAL 3 – TIME: _____

Most likely too many carbs
- ☐ Headache
- ☐ Anxiety
- ☐ Jittery/wired
- ☐ Difficulty concentrating
- ☐ Hunger is not satisfied
- ☐ Crave sweet
- ☐ Crave Protein & fat

Balanced Responses
- ☐ Appetite feels satisfied
- ☐ Feel emotionally balanced
- ☐ Good mental focus
- ☐ Normal level of energy
- ☐ No cravings for sweets
- ☐ No cravings for more food

Most likely too much protein &/or fat
- ☐ Lethargic
- ☐ Mentally Sluggish
- ☐ Heavy Gut
- ☐ Feel full yet still hungry
- ☐ Crave sweets
- ☐ Crave Caffeine
(if more than hour after meal could be a crash from too much carb)

Approx. of macro Nutrient ratios of meal
% Carbs _____
% Protein _____
% Fat _____
Foods Eaten: _____
_____
_____
_____
_____

SNACKS:

Time: _____ Details: _____
Time: _____ Details: _____
Time: _____ Details: _____

DRINKS:

Details: _____
_____
_____

LIFESTYLE:

What time did you go to sleep?_____ What time did you get up? _____

Sleep quality? ☐ Sound ☐ Restless   Did you have night Sweats? ☐ Yes ☐ No

Did you awake during night (give time & reason)? _____

Did you wake up refreshed today or tired? ☐ Refreshed ☐ Tired

Did you start slow this morning? ☐ Yes ☐ No   If yes, how long did it take to feel alert? _____

Bowel movement(s)?
(number, colour, size & shape)
_____
_____

MOVEMENT :

Details: _____
_____
_____

GENERAL:

How did you feel today? _____
_____
_____

OTHER INFO: _____

DAILY FOOD & LIFESTYLE DIARY

DAILY FOOD DIARY - DATE: _____

Complete everyday for 12 weeks

Please fill out form 1-2 hours after each meal

MEAL 1 – TIME: _____

Most likely too many carbs

- ☐ Headache
- ☐ Anxiety
- ☐ Jittery/wired
- ☐ Difficulty concentrating
- ☐ Hunger is not satisfied
- ☐ Crave sweet
- ☐ Crave Protein & fat

Balanced Responses

- ☐ Appetite feels satisfied
- ☐ Feel emotionally balanced
- ☐ Good mental focus
- ☐ Normal level of energy
- ☐ No cravings for sweets
- ☐ No cravings for more food

Most likely too much protein &/or fat

- ☐ Lethargic
- ☐ Mentally Sluggish
- ☐ Heavy Gut
- ☐ Feel full yet still hungry
- ☐ Crave sweets
- ☐ Crave Caffeine

(if more than hour after meal could be a crash from too much carb)

Approx. of macro Nutrient ratios of meal
% Carbs _____
% Protein _____
% Fat _____
Foods Eaten: _____
_____
_____
_____
_____
_____

MEAL 2 – TIME: _____

Most likely too many carbs

- ☐ Headache
- ☐ Anxiety
- ☐ Jittery/wired
- ☐ Difficulty concentrating
- ☐ Hunger is not satisfied
- ☐ Crave sweet
- ☐ Crave Protein & fat

Balanced Responses

- ☐ Appetite feels satisfied
- ☐ Feel emotionally balanced
- ☐ Good mental focus
- ☐ Normal level of energy
- ☐ No cravings for sweets
- ☐ No cravings for more food

Most likely too much protein &/or fat

- ☐ Lethargic
- ☐ Mentally Sluggish
- ☐ Heavy Gut
- ☐ Feel full yet still hungry
- ☐ Crave sweets
- ☐ Crave Caffeine

(if more than hour after meal could be a crash from too much carb)

Approx. of macro Nutrient ratios of meal
% Carbs _____
% Protein _____
% Fat _____
Foods Eaten: _____
_____
_____
_____
_____
_____

MEAL 3 – TIME: _____

Most likely too many carbs

- ☐ Headache
- ☐ Anxiety
- ☐ Jittery/wired
- ☐ Difficulty concentrating
- ☐ Hunger is not satisfied
- ☐ Crave sweet
- ☐ Crave Protein & fat

Balanced Responses

- ☐ Appetite feels satisfied
- ☐ Feel emotionally balanced
- ☐ Good mental focus
- ☐ Normal level of energy
- ☐ No cravings for sweets
- ☐ No cravings for more food

Most likely too much protein &/or fat

- ☐ Lethargic
- ☐ Mentally Sluggish
- ☐ Heavy Gut
- ☐ Feel full yet still hungry
- ☐ Crave sweets
- ☐ Crave Caffeine

(if more than hour after meal could be a crash from too much carb)

Approx. of macro Nutrient ratios of meal
% Carbs _____
% Protein _____
% Fat _____
Foods Eaten: _____
_____
_____
_____
_____

SNACKS:

Time: _____ Details: _____
Time: _____ Details: _____
Time: _____ Details: _____

DRINKS:

Details: _____
_____
_____

LIFESTYLE:

What time did you go to sleep?_____ What time did you get up? _____

Sleep quality? ☐ Sound ☐ Restless   Did you have night Sweats? ☐ Yes ☐ No

Did you awake during night (give time & reason)? _____

Did you wake up refreshed today or tired? ☐ Refreshed ☐ Tired

Did you start slow this morning? ☐ Yes ☐ No   If yes, how long did it take to feel alert? _____

Bowel movement(s)?
(number, colour, size & shape)
_____
_____

MOVEMENT :

Details: _____
_____
_____

GENERAL:

How did you feel today? _____
_____
_____

OTHER INFO: _____

DAILY FOOD & LIFESTYLE DIARY

DAILY FOOD DIARY - DATE: _____

Complete everyday for 12 weeks

Please fill out form 1-2 hours after each meal

MEAL 1 – TIME: _____

Most likely too many carbs	Balanced Responses	Most likely too much protein &/or fat	
☐ Headache	☐ Appetite feels satisfied	☐ Lethargic	Approx. of macro Nutrient ratios of meal
☐ Anxiety	☐ Feel emotionally balanced	☐ Mentally Sluggish	% Carbs _____
☐ Jittery/wired	☐ Good mental focus	☐ Heavy Gut	% Protein _____
☐ Difficulty concentrating	☐ Normal level of energy	☐ Feel full yet still hungry	% Fat _____
☐ Hunger is not satisfied	☐ No cravings for sweets	☐ Crave sweets	Foods Eaten: _____
☐ Crave sweet	☐ No cravings for more food	☐ Crave Caffeine	
☐ Crave Protein & fat		(if more than hour after meal could be a crash from too much carb)	

MEAL 2 – TIME: _____

Most likely too many carbs	Balanced Responses	Most likely too much protein &/or fat	
☐ Headache	☐ Appetite feels satisfied	☐ Lethargic	Approx. of macro Nutrient ratios of meal
☐ Anxiety	☐ Feel emotionally balanced	☐ Mentally Sluggish	% Carbs _____
☐ Jittery/wired	☐ Good mental focus	☐ Heavy Gut	% Protein _____
☐ Difficulty concentrating	☐ Normal level of energy	☐ Feel full yet still hungry	% Fat _____
☐ Hunger is not satisfied	☐ No cravings for sweets	☐ Crave sweets	Foods Eaten: _____
☐ Crave sweet	☐ No cravings for more food	☐ Crave Caffeine	
☐ Crave Protein & fat		(if more than hour after meal could be a crash from too much carb)	

MEAL 3 – TIME: _____

Most likely too many carbs	Balanced Responses	Most likely too much protein &/or fat	
☐ Headache	☐ Appetite feels satisfied	☐ Lethargic	Approx. of macro Nutrient ratios of meal
☐ Anxiety	☐ Feel emotionally balanced	☐ Mentally Sluggish	% Carbs _____
☐ Jittery/wired	☐ Good mental focus	☐ Heavy Gut	% Protein _____
☐ Difficulty concentrating	☐ Normal level of energy	☐ Feel full yet still hungry	% Fat _____
☐ Hunger is not satisfied	☐ No cravings for sweets	☐ Crave sweets	Foods Eaten: _____
☐ Crave sweet	☐ No cravings for more food	☐ Crave Caffeine	
☐ Crave Protein & fat		(if more than hour after meal could be a crash from too much carb)	

SNACKS:

Time: _____ Details: _____
Time: _____ Details: _____
Time: _____ Details: _____

DRINKS:

Details: _____
_____
_____

LIFESTYLE:

What time did you go to sleep? _____ What time did you get up? _____
Sleep quality? ☐ Sound ☐ Restless Did you have night Sweats? ☐ Yes ☐ No
Did you awake during night (give time & reason)? _____
Did you wake up refreshed today or tired? ☐ Refreshed ☐ Tired
Did you start slow this morning? ☐ Yes ☐ No If yes, how long did it take to feel alert? _____

Bowel movement(s)?
(number, colour, size & shape)
_____
_____

MOVEMENT :

Details: _____
_____
_____

GENERAL:

How did you feel today? _____
_____
_____

OTHER INFO: _____

DAILY FOOD & LIFESTYLE DIARY

DAILY FOOD DIARY - DATE: _____

Complete everyday for 12 weeks

MEAL 1 – TIME: _____

Please fill out form 1-2 hours after each meal

Most likely too many carbs

- ☐ Headache
- ☐ Anxiety
- ☐ Jittery/wired
- ☐ Difficulty concentrating
- ☐ Hunger is not satisfied
- ☐ Crave sweet
- ☐ Crave Protein & fat

Balanced Responses

- ☐ Appetite feels satisfied
- ☐ Feel emotionally balanced
- ☐ Good mental focus
- ☐ Normal level of energy
- ☐ No cravings for sweets
- ☐ No cravings for more food

Most likely too much protein &/or fat

- ☐ Lethargic
- ☐ Mentally Sluggish
- ☐ Heavy Gut
- ☐ Feel full yet still hungry
- ☐ Crave sweets
- ☐ Crave Caffeine

(if more than hour after meal could be a crash from too much carb)

Approx. of macro Nutrient ratios of meal
% Carbs _____
% Protein _____
% Fat _____
Foods Eaten: _____
_____
_____
_____
_____
_____

MEAL 2 – TIME: _____

Most likely too many carbs

- ☐ Headache
- ☐ Anxiety
- ☐ Jittery/wired
- ☐ Difficulty concentrating
- ☐ Hunger is not satisfied
- ☐ Crave sweet
- ☐ Crave Protein & fat

Balanced Responses

- ☐ Appetite feels satisfied
- ☐ Feel emotionally balanced
- ☐ Good mental focus
- ☐ Normal level of energy
- ☐ No cravings for sweets
- ☐ No cravings for more food

Most likely too much protein &/or fat

- ☐ Lethargic
- ☐ Mentally Sluggish
- ☐ Heavy Gut
- ☐ Feel full yet still hungry
- ☐ Crave sweets
- ☐ Crave Caffeine

(if more than hour after meal could be a crash from too much carb)

Approx. of macro Nutrient ratios of meal
% Carbs _____
% Protein _____
% Fat _____
Foods Eaten: _____
_____
_____
_____
_____
_____

MEAL 3 – TIME: _____

Most likely too many carbs

- ☐ Headache
- ☐ Anxiety
- ☐ Jittery/wired
- ☐ Difficulty concentrating
- ☐ Hunger is not satisfied
- ☐ Crave sweet
- ☐ Crave Protein & fat

Balanced Responses

- ☐ Appetite feels satisfied
- ☐ Feel emotionally balanced
- ☐ Good mental focus
- ☐ Normal level of energy
- ☐ No cravings for sweets
- ☐ No cravings for more food

Most likely too much protein &/or fat

- ☐ Lethargic
- ☐ Mentally Sluggish
- ☐ Heavy Gut
- ☐ Feel full yet still hungry
- ☐ Crave sweets
- ☐ Crave Caffeine

(if more than hour after meal could be a crash from too much carb)

Approx. of macro Nutrient ratios of meal
% Carbs _____
% Protein _____
% Fat _____
Foods Eaten: _____
_____
_____
_____
_____
_____

SNACKS:

Time: _____ Details: _____
Time: _____ Details: _____
Time: _____ Details: _____

DRINKS:

Details: _____
_____
_____

LIFESTYLE:

What time did you go to sleep? _____ What time did you get up? _____
Sleep quality? ☐ Sound ☐ Restless   Did you have night Sweats? ☐ Yes ☐ No
Did you awake during night (give time & reason)? _____
Did you wake up refreshed today or tired? ☐ Refreshed ☐ Tired
Did you start slow this morning? ☐ Yes ☐ No   If yes, how long did it take to feel alert? _____

Bowel movement(s)?
(number, colour, size & shape)
_____
_____

MOVEMENT :

Details: _____
_____
_____

GENERAL:

How did you feel today? _____
_____
_____

OTHER INFO: _____

DAILY FOOD & LIFESTYLE DIARY

DAILY FOOD DIARY - DATE: _____

Complete everyday for 12 weeks

MEAL 1 – TIME: _____

Please fill out form 1-2 hours after each meal

Most likely too many carbs	Balanced Responses	Most likely too much protein &/or fat	
☐ Headache	☐ Appetite feels satisfied	☐ Lethargic	Approx. of macro Nutrient ratios of meal
☐ Anxiety	☐ Feel emotionally balanced	☐ Mentally Sluggish	% Carbs _____
☐ Jittery/wired	☐ Good mental focus	☐ Heavy Gut	% Protein _____
☐ Difficulty concentrating	☐ Normal level of energy	☐ Feel full yet still hungry	% Fat _____
☐ Hunger is not satisfied	☐ No cravings for sweets	☐ Crave sweets	Foods Eaten: _____
☐ Crave sweet	☐ No cravings for more food	☐ Crave Caffeine	_____
☐ Crave Protein & fat		(if more than hour after meal could	_____
		be a crash from too much carb)	_____

MEAL 2 – TIME: _____

Most likely too many carbs	Balanced Responses	Most likely too much protein &/or fat	
☐ Headache	☐ Appetite feels satisfied	☐ Lethargic	Approx. of macro Nutrient ratios of meal
☐ Anxiety	☐ Feel emotionally balanced	☐ Mentally Sluggish	% Carbs _____
☐ Jittery/wired	☐ Good mental focus	☐ Heavy Gut	% Protein _____
☐ Difficulty concentrating	☐ Normal level of energy	☐ Feel full yet still hungry	% Fat _____
☐ Hunger is not satisfied	☐ No cravings for sweets	☐ Crave sweets	Foods Eaten: _____
☐ Crave sweet	☐ No cravings for more food	☐ Crave Caffeine	_____
☐ Crave Protein & fat		(if more than hour after meal could	_____
		be a crash from too much carb)	_____

MEAL 3 – TIME: _____

Most likely too many carbs	Balanced Responses	Most likely too much protein &/or fat	
☐ Headache	☐ Appetite feels satisfied	☐ Lethargic	Approx. of macro Nutrient ratios of meal
☐ Anxiety	☐ Feel emotionally balanced	☐ Mentally Sluggish	% Carbs _____
☐ Jittery/wired	☐ Good mental focus	☐ Heavy Gut	% Protein _____
☐ Difficulty concentrating	☐ Normal level of energy	☐ Feel full yet still hungry	% Fat _____
☐ Hunger is not satisfied	☐ No cravings for sweets	☐ Crave sweets	Foods Eaten: _____
☐ Crave sweet	☐ No cravings for more food	☐ Crave Caffeine	_____
☐ Crave Protein & fat		(if more than hour after meal could	_____
		be a crash from too much carb)	_____

SNACKS:

Time: _____ Details: _____
Time: _____ Details: _____
Time: _____ Details: _____

DRINKS:

Details: _____
_____
_____

LIFESTYLE:

What time did you go to sleep? _____ What time did you get up? _____

Bowel movement(s)?
(number, colour, size & shape)

Sleep quality? ☐ Sound ☐ Restless   Did you have night Sweats? ☐ Yes ☐ No

Did you awake during night (give time & reason)? _____

Did you wake up refreshed today or tired? ☐ Refreshed ☐ Tired

Did you start slow this morning? ☐ Yes ☐ No   If yes, how long did it take to feel alert? _____

MOVEMENT :

Details: _____
_____
_____

GENERAL:

How did you feel today? _____
_____
_____

OTHER INFO: _____

DAILY FOOD & LIFESTYLE DIARY

DAILY FOOD DIARY - DATE: _____

MEAL 1 – TIME: _____

Complete everyday for 12 weeks

Please fill out form 1-2 hours after each meal

Most likely too many carbs

☐ Headache
☐ Anxiety
☐ Jittery/wired
☐ Difficulty concentrating
☐ Hunger is not satisfied
☐ Crave sweet
☐ Crave Protein & fat

Balanced Responses

☐ Appetite feels satisfied
☐ Feel emotionally balanced
☐ Good mental focus
☐ Normal level of energy
☐ No cravings for sweets
☐ No cravings for more food

Most likely too much protein &/or fat

☐ Lethargic
☐ Mentally Sluggish
☐ Heavy Gut
☐ Feel full yet still hungry
☐ Crave sweets
☐ Crave Caffeine
(if more than hour after meal could
be a crash from too much carb)

Approx. of macro Nutrient ratios of meal
% Carbs _____
% Protein _____
% Fat _____
Foods Eaten: _____
_____
_____
_____
_____
_____

MEAL 2 – TIME: _____

Most likely too many carbs

☐ Headache
☐ Anxiety
☐ Jittery/wired
☐ Difficulty concentrating
☐ Hunger is not satisfied
☐ Crave sweet
☐ Crave Protein & fat

Balanced Responses

☐ Appetite feels satisfied
☐ Feel emotionally balanced
☐ Good mental focus
☐ Normal level of energy
☐ No cravings for sweets
☐ No cravings for more food

Most likely too much protein &/or fat

☐ Lethargic
☐ Mentally Sluggish
☐ Heavy Gut
☐ Feel full yet still hungry
☐ Crave sweets
☐ Crave Caffeine
(if more than hour after meal could
be a crash from too much carb)

Approx. of macro Nutrient ratios of meal
% Carbs _____
% Protein _____
% Fat _____
Foods Eaten: _____
_____
_____
_____
_____
_____

MEAL 3 – TIME: _____

Most likely too many carbs

☐ Headache
☐ Anxiety
☐ Jittery/wired
☐ Difficulty concentrating
☐ Hunger is not satisfied
☐ Crave sweet
☐ Crave Protein & fat

Balanced Responses

☐ Appetite feels satisfied
☐ Feel emotionally balanced
☐ Good mental focus
☐ Normal level of energy
☐ No cravings for sweets
☐ No cravings for more food

Most likely too much protein &/or fat

☐ Lethargic
☐ Mentally Sluggish
☐ Heavy Gut
☐ Feel full yet still hungry
☐ Crave sweets
☐ Crave Caffeine
(if more than hour after meal could
be a crash from too much carb)

Approx. of macro Nutrient ratios of meal
% Carbs _____
% Protein _____
% Fat _____
Foods Eaten: _____
_____
_____
_____
_____
_____

SNACKS:

Time: _____ Details: _____
Time: _____ Details: _____
Time: _____ Details: _____

DRINKS:

Details: _____
_____
_____

LIFESTYLE:

What time did you go to sleep? _____ What time did you get up? _____
Sleep quality? ☐ Sound ☐ Restless   Did you have night Sweats? ☐ Yes ☐ No
Did you awake during night (give time & reason)? _____
Did you wake up refreshed today or tired? ☐ Refreshed ☐ Tired
Did you start slow this morning? ☐ Yes ☐ No   If yes, how long did it take to feel alert? _____

Bowel movement(s)?
(number, colour, size & shape)
_____
_____

MOVEMENT :

Details: _____
_____
_____

GENERAL:

How did you feel today? _____
_____
_____

OTHER INFO: _____

DAILY FOOD & LIFESTYLE DIARY

DAILY FOOD DIARY - DATE: _____

Complete everyday for 12 weeks

Please fill out form 1-2 hours after each meal

MEAL 1 – TIME: _____

Most likely too many carbs	Balanced Responses	Most likely too much protein &/or fat	Approx. of macro Nutrient ratios of meal
☐ Headache	☐ Appetite feels satisfied	☐ Lethargic	% Carbs _____
☐ Anxiety	☐ Feel emotionally balanced	☐ Mentally Sluggish	% Protein _____
☐ Jittery/wired	☐ Good mental focus	☐ Heavy Gut	% Fat _____
☐ Difficulty concentrating	☐ Normal level of energy	☐ Feel full yet still hungry	Foods Eaten: _____
☐ Hunger is not satisfied	☐ No cravings for sweets	☐ Crave sweets	_____
☐ Crave sweet	☐ No cravings for more food	☐ Crave Caffeine	_____
☐ Crave Protein & fat		(if more than hour after meal could be a crash from too much carb)	_____

MEAL 2 – TIME: _____

Most likely too many carbs	Balanced Responses	Most likely too much protein &/or fat	Approx. of macro Nutrient ratios of meal
☐ Headache	☐ Appetite feels satisfied	☐ Lethargic	% Carbs _____
☐ Anxiety	☐ Feel emotionally balanced	☐ Mentally Sluggish	% Protein _____
☐ Jittery/wired	☐ Good mental focus	☐ Heavy Gut	% Fat _____
☐ Difficulty concentrating	☐ Normal level of energy	☐ Feel full yet still hungry	Foods Eaten: _____
☐ Hunger is not satisfied	☐ No cravings for sweets	☐ Crave sweets	_____
☐ Crave sweet	☐ No cravings for more food	☐ Crave Caffeine	_____
☐ Crave Protein & fat		(if more than hour after meal could be a crash from too much carb)	_____

MEAL 3 – TIME: _____

Most likely too many carbs	Balanced Responses	Most likely too much protein &/or fat	Approx. of macro Nutrient ratios of meal
☐ Headache	☐ Appetite feels satisfied	☐ Lethargic	% Carbs _____
☐ Anxiety	☐ Feel emotionally balanced	☐ Mentally Sluggish	% Protein _____
☐ Jittery/wired	☐ Good mental focus	☐ Heavy Gut	% Fat _____
☐ Difficulty concentrating	☐ Normal level of energy	☐ Feel full yet still hungry	Foods Eaten: _____
☐ Hunger is not satisfied	☐ No cravings for sweets	☐ Crave sweets	_____
☐ Crave sweet	☐ No cravings for more food	☐ Crave Caffeine	_____
☐ Crave Protein & fat		(if more than hour after meal could be a crash from too much carb)	_____

SNACKS:

Time: _____ Details: _____
Time: _____ Details: _____
Time: _____ Details: _____

DRINKS:

Details: _____
_____
_____

LIFESTYLE:

What time did you go to sleep? _____ What time did you get up? _____ Bowel movement(s)? (number, colour, size & shape)
Sleep quality? ☐ Sound ☐ Restless   Did you have night Sweats? ☐ Yes ☐ No
Did you awake during night (give time & reason)? _____
Did you wake up refreshed today or tired? ☐ Refreshed ☐ Tired
Did you start slow this morning? ☐ Yes ☐ No   If yes, how long did it take to feel alert? _____

MOVEMENT :

Details: _____

GENERAL:

How did you feel today? _____

OTHER INFO: _____

DAILY FOOD & LIFESTYLE DIARY

DAILY FOOD DIARY - DATE: _____

Complete everyday for 12 weeks

Please fill out form 1-2 hours after each meal

MEAL 1 – TIME: _____

Most likely too many carbs

- ☐ Headache
- ☐ Anxiety
- ☐ Jittery/wired
- ☐ Difficulty concentrating
- ☐ Hunger is not satisfied
- ☐ Crave sweet
- ☐ Crave Protein & fat

Balanced Responses

- ☐ Appetite feels satisfied
- ☐ Feel emotionally balanced
- ☐ Good mental focus
- ☐ Normal level of energy
- ☐ No cravings for sweets
- ☐ No cravings for more food

Most likely too much protein &/or fat

- ☐ Lethargic
- ☐ Mentally Sluggish
- ☐ Heavy Gut
- ☐ Feel full yet still hungry
- ☐ Crave sweets
- ☐ Crave Caffeine
(if more than hour after meal could be a crash from too much carb)

Approx. of macro Nutrient ratios of meal
% Carbs _____
% Protein _____
% Fat _____
Foods Eaten: _____
_____
_____
_____
_____
_____

MEAL 2 – TIME: _____

Most likely too many carbs

- ☐ Headache
- ☐ Anxiety
- ☐ Jittery/wired
- ☐ Difficulty concentrating
- ☐ Hunger is not satisfied
- ☐ Crave sweet
- ☐ Crave Protein & fat

Balanced Responses

- ☐ Appetite feels satisfied
- ☐ Feel emotionally balanced
- ☐ Good mental focus
- ☐ Normal level of energy
- ☐ No cravings for sweets
- ☐ No cravings for more food

Most likely too much protein &/or fat

- ☐ Lethargic
- ☐ Mentally Sluggish
- ☐ Heavy Gut
- ☐ Feel full yet still hungry
- ☐ Crave sweets
- ☐ Crave Caffeine
(if more than hour after meal could be a crash from too much carb)

Approx. of macro Nutrient ratios of meal
% Carbs _____
% Protein _____
% Fat _____
Foods Eaten: _____
_____
_____
_____
_____

MEAL 3 – TIME: _____

Most likely too many carbs

- ☐ Headache
- ☐ Anxiety
- ☐ Jittery/wired
- ☐ Difficulty concentrating
- ☐ Hunger is not satisfied
- ☐ Crave sweet
- ☐ Crave Protein & fat

Balanced Responses

- ☐ Appetite feels satisfied
- ☐ Feel emotionally balanced
- ☐ Good mental focus
- ☐ Normal level of energy
- ☐ No cravings for sweets
- ☐ No cravings for more food

Most likely too much protein &/or fat

- ☐ Lethargic
- ☐ Mentally Sluggish
- ☐ Heavy Gut
- ☐ Feel full yet still hungry
- ☐ Crave sweets
- ☐ Crave Caffeine
(if more than hour after meal could be a crash from too much carb)

Approx. of macro Nutrient ratios of meal
% Carbs _____
% Protein _____
% Fat _____
Foods Eaten: _____
_____
_____
_____
_____
_____

SNACKS:

Time: _____ Details: _____
Time: _____ Details: _____
Time: _____ Details: _____

DRINKS:

Details: _____
_____
_____

LIFESTYLE:

What time did you go to sleep? _____ What time did you get up? _____
Sleep quality? ☐ Sound ☐ Restless Did you have night Sweats? ☐ Yes ☐ No
Did you awake during night (give time & reason)? _____
Did you wake up refreshed today or tired? ☐ Refreshed ☐ Tired
Did you start slow this morning? ☐ Yes ☐ No   If yes, how long did it take to feel alert? _____

Bowel movement(s)?
(number, colour, size & shape)
_____
_____

MOVEMENT :

Details: _____
_____
_____

GENERAL:

How did you feel today? _____
_____

OTHER INFO: _____

DAILY FOOD & LIFESTYLE DIARY

DAILY FOOD DIARY - DATE: _____

Complete everyday for 12 weeks

MEAL 1 – TIME: _____

Please fill out form 1-2 hours after each meal

Most likely too many carbs
- ☐ Headache
- ☐ Anxiety
- ☐ Jittery/wired
- ☐ Difficulty concentrating
- ☐ Hunger is not satisfied
- ☐ Crave sweet
- ☐ Crave Protein & fat

Balanced Responses
- ☐ Appetite feels satisfied
- ☐ Feel emotionally balanced
- ☐ Good mental focus
- ☐ Normal level of energy
- ☐ No cravings for sweets
- ☐ No cravings for more food

Most likely too much protein &/or fat
- ☐ Lethargic
- ☐ Mentally Sluggish
- ☐ Heavy Gut
- ☐ Feel full yet still hungry
- ☐ Crave sweets
- ☐ Crave Caffeine
(if more than hour after meal could be a crash from too much carb)

Approx. of macro Nutrient ratios of meal
% Carbs _____
% Protein _____
% Fat _____
Foods Eaten: _____
_____
_____
_____
_____
_____
_____

MEAL 2 – TIME: _____

Most likely too many carbs
- ☐ Headache
- ☐ Anxiety
- ☐ Jittery/wired
- ☐ Difficulty concentrating
- ☐ Hunger is not satisfied
- ☐ Crave sweet
- ☐ Crave Protein & fat

Balanced Responses
- ☐ Appetite feels satisfied
- ☐ Feel emotionally balanced
- ☐ Good mental focus
- ☐ Normal level of energy
- ☐ No cravings for sweets
- ☐ No cravings for more food

Most likely too much protein &/or fat
- ☐ Lethargic
- ☐ Mentally Sluggish
- ☐ Heavy Gut
- ☐ Feel full yet still hungry
- ☐ Crave sweets
- ☐ Crave Caffeine
(if more than hour after meal could be a crash from too much carb)

Approx. of macro Nutrient ratios of meal
% Carbs _____
% Protein _____
% Fat _____
Foods Eaten: _____
_____
_____
_____
_____
_____
_____

MEAL 3 – TIME: _____

Most likely too many carbs
- ☐ Headache
- ☐ Anxiety
- ☐ Jittery/wired
- ☐ Difficulty concentrating
- ☐ Hunger is not satisfied
- ☐ Crave sweet
- ☐ Crave Protein & fat

Balanced Responses
- ☐ Appetite feels satisfied
- ☐ Feel emotionally balanced
- ☐ Good mental focus
- ☐ Normal level of energy
- ☐ No cravings for sweets
- ☐ No cravings for more food

Most likely too much protein &/or fat
- ☐ Lethargic
- ☐ Mentally Sluggish
- ☐ Heavy Gut
- ☐ Feel full yet still hungry
- ☐ Crave sweets
- ☐ Crave Caffeine
(if more than hour after meal could be a crash from too much carb)

Approx. of macro Nutrient ratios of meal
% Carbs _____
% Protein _____
% Fat _____
Foods Eaten: _____
_____
_____
_____
_____
_____
_____

SNACKS:

Time: _____ Details: _____
Time: _____ Details: _____
Time: _____ Details: _____

DRINKS:

Details: _____
_____
_____

LIFESTYLE:

What time did you go to sleep? _____ What time did you get up? _____ Bowel movement(s)?
Sleep quality? ☐ Sound ☐ Restless   Did you have night Sweats? ☐ Yes ☐ No   (number, colour, size & shape)
Did you awake during night (give time & reason)? _____
Did you wake up refreshed today or tired? ☐ Refreshed ☐ Tired
Did you start slow this morning? ☐ Yes ☐ No   If yes, how long did it take to feel alert? _____

MOVEMENT :

Details: _____
_____
_____

GENERAL:

How did you feel today? _____
_____
_____

OTHER INFO: _____

DAILY FOOD & LIFESTYLE DIARY

DAILY FOOD DIARY - DATE: _____

Complete everyday for 12 weeks

Please fill out form 1-2 hours after each meal

MEAL 1 – TIME: _____

Most likely too many carbs

- ☐ Headache
- ☐ Anxiety
- ☐ Jittery/wired
- ☐ Difficulty concentrating
- ☐ Hunger is not satisfied
- ☐ Crave sweet
- ☐ Crave Protein & fat

Balanced Responses

- ☐ Appetite feels satisfied
- ☐ Feel emotionally balanced
- ☐ Good mental focus
- ☐ Normal level of energy
- ☐ No cravings for sweets
- ☐ No cravings for more food

Most likely too much protein &/or fat

- ☐ Lethargic
- ☐ Mentally Sluggish
- ☐ Heavy Gut
- ☐ Feel full yet still hungry
- ☐ Crave sweets
- ☐ Crave Caffeine

(if more than hour after meal could be a crash from too much carb)

Approx. of macro Nutrient ratios of meal

% Carbs _____
% Protein _____
% Fat _____
Foods Eaten: _____
_____
_____
_____
_____

MEAL 2 – TIME: _____

Most likely too many carbs

- ☐ Headache
- ☐ Anxiety
- ☐ Jittery/wired
- ☐ Difficulty concentrating
- ☐ Hunger is not satisfied
- ☐ Crave sweet
- ☐ Crave Protein & fat

Balanced Responses

- ☐ Appetite feels satisfied
- ☐ Feel emotionally balanced
- ☐ Good mental focus
- ☐ Normal level of energy
- ☐ No cravings for sweets
- ☐ No cravings for more food

Most likely too much protein &/or fat

- ☐ Lethargic
- ☐ Mentally Sluggish
- ☐ Heavy Gut
- ☐ Feel full yet still hungry
- ☐ Crave sweets
- ☐ Crave Caffeine

(if more than hour after meal could be a crash from too much carb)

Approx. of macro Nutrient ratios of meal

% Carbs _____
% Protein _____
% Fat _____
Foods Eaten: _____
_____
_____
_____
_____

MEAL 3 – TIME: _____

Most likely too many carbs

- ☐ Headache
- ☐ Anxiety
- ☐ Jittery/wired
- ☐ Difficulty concentrating
- ☐ Hunger is not satisfied
- ☐ Crave sweet
- ☐ Crave Protein & fat

Balanced Responses

- ☐ Appetite feels satisfied
- ☐ Feel emotionally balanced
- ☐ Good mental focus
- ☐ Normal level of energy
- ☐ No cravings for sweets
- ☐ No cravings for more food

Most likely too much protein &/or fat

- ☐ Lethargic
- ☐ Mentally Sluggish
- ☐ Heavy Gut
- ☐ Feel full yet still hungry
- ☐ Crave sweets
- ☐ Crave Caffeine

(if more than hour after meal could be a crash from too much carb)

Approx. of macro Nutrient ratios of meal

% Carbs _____
% Protein _____
% Fat _____
Foods Eaten: _____
_____
_____
_____
_____

SNACKS:

Time: _____ Details: _____
Time: _____ Details: _____
Time: _____ Details: _____

DRINKS:

Details: _____
_____
_____

LIFESTYLE:

What time did you go to sleep? _____   What time did you get up? _____
Sleep quality? ☐ Sound ☐ Restless   Did you have night Sweats? ☐ Yes ☐ No
Did you awake during night (give time & reason)? _____
Did you wake up refreshed today or tired? ☐ Refreshed ☐ Tired
Did you start slow this morning? ☐ Yes ☐ No   If yes, how long did it take to feel alert? _____

Bowel movement(s)?
(number, colour, size & shape)
_____
_____

MOVEMENT :

Details: _____
_____
_____

GENERAL:

How did you feel today? _____
_____
_____

OTHER INFO: _____

DAILY FOOD & LIFESTYLE DIARY

DAILY FOOD DIARY - DATE: _____

Complete everyday for 12 weeks

MEAL 1 – TIME: _____

Please fill out form 1-2 hours after each meal

Most likely too many carbs

☐ Headache
☐ Anxiety
☐ Jittery/wired
☐ Difficulty concentrating
☐ Hunger is not satisfied
☐ Crave sweet
☐ Crave Protein & fat

Balanced Responses

☐ Appetite feels satisfied
☐ Feel emotionally balanced
☐ Good mental focus
☐ Normal level of energy
☐ No cravings for sweets
☐ No cravings for more food

Most likely too much protein &/or fat

☐ Lethargic
☐ Mentally Sluggish
☐ Heavy Gut
☐ Feel full yet still hungry
☐ Crave sweets
☐ Crave Caffeine
(if more than hour after meal could
be a crash from too much carb)

Approx. of macro Nutrient ratios of meal
% Carbs _____
% Protein _____
% Fat _____
Foods Eaten: _____
_____
_____
_____
_____
_____

MEAL 2 – TIME: _____

Most likely too many carbs

☐ Headache
☐ Anxiety
☐ Jittery/wired
☐ Difficulty concentrating
☐ Hunger is not satisfied
☐ Crave sweet
☐ Crave Protein & fat

Balanced Responses

☐ Appetite feels satisfied
☐ Feel emotionally balanced
☐ Good mental focus
☐ Normal level of energy
☐ No cravings for sweets
☐ No cravings for more food

Most likely too much protein &/or fat

☐ Lethargic
☐ Mentally Sluggish
☐ Heavy Gut
☐ Feel full yet still hungry
☐ Crave sweets
☐ Crave Caffeine
(if more than hour after meal could
be a crash from too much carb)

Approx. of macro Nutrient ratios of meal
% Carbs _____
% Protein _____
% Fat _____
Foods Eaten: _____
_____
_____
_____
_____
_____

MEAL 3 – TIME: _____

Most likely too many carbs

☐ Headache
☐ Anxiety
☐ Jittery/wired
☐ Difficulty concentrating
☐ Hunger is not satisfied
☐ Crave sweet
☐ Crave Protein & fat

Balanced Responses

☐ Appetite feels satisfied
☐ Feel emotionally balanced
☐ Good mental focus
☐ Normal level of energy
☐ No cravings for sweets
☐ No cravings for more food

Most likely too much protein &/or fat

☐ Lethargic
☐ Mentally Sluggish
☐ Heavy Gut
☐ Feel full yet still hungry
☐ Crave sweets
☐ Crave Caffeine
(if more than hour after meal could
be a crash from too much carb)

Approx. of macro Nutrient ratios of meal
% Carbs _____
% Protein _____
% Fat _____
Foods Eaten: _____
_____
_____
_____
_____

SNACKS:

Time: _____ Details: _____
Time: _____ Details: _____
Time: _____ Details: _____

DRINKS:

Details: _____
_____
_____

LIFESTYLE:

What time did you go to sleep? _____ What time did you get up? _____

Sleep quality? ☐ Sound ☐ Restless   Did you have night Sweats? ☐ Yes ☐ No

Did you awake during night (give time & reason)? _____

Did you wake up refreshed today or tired? ☐ Refreshed ☐ Tired

Did you start slow this morning? ☐ Yes ☐ No   If yes, how long did it take to feel alert? _____

Bowel movement(s)?
(number, colour, size & shape)
_____
_____

MOVEMENT :

Details: _____
_____
_____

GENERAL:

How did you feel today? _____
_____
_____

OTHER INFO: _____

DAILY FOOD & LIFESTYLE DIARY

DAILY FOOD DIARY - DATE: _____

Complete everyday for 12 weeks

MEAL 1 – TIME: _____

Please fill out form 1-2 hours after each meal

Most likely too many carbs

- ☐ Headache
- ☐ Anxiety
- ☐ Jittery/wired
- ☐ Difficulty concentrating
- ☐ Hunger is not satisfied
- ☐ Crave sweet
- ☐ Crave Protein & fat

Balanced Responses

- ☐ Appetite feels satisfied
- ☐ Feel emotionally balanced
- ☐ Good mental focus
- ☐ Normal level of energy
- ☐ No cravings for sweets
- ☐ No cravings for more food

Most likely too much protein &/or fat

- ☐ Lethargic
- ☐ Mentally Sluggish
- ☐ Heavy Gut
- ☐ Feel full yet still hungry
- ☐ Crave sweets
- ☐ Crave Caffeine

(if more than hour after meal could be a crash from too much carb)

Approx. of macro Nutrient ratios of meal

% Carbs _____
% Protein _____
% Fat _____
Foods Eaten: _____
_____
_____
_____
_____
_____

MEAL 2 – TIME: _____

Most likely too many carbs

- ☐ Headache
- ☐ Anxiety
- ☐ Jittery/wired
- ☐ Difficulty concentrating
- ☐ Hunger is not satisfied
- ☐ Crave sweet
- ☐ Crave Protein & fat

Balanced Responses

- ☐ Appetite feels satisfied
- ☐ Feel emotionally balanced
- ☐ Good mental focus
- ☐ Normal level of energy
- ☐ No cravings for sweets
- ☐ No cravings for more food

Most likely too much protein &/or fat

- ☐ Lethargic
- ☐ Mentally Sluggish
- ☐ Heavy Gut
- ☐ Feel full yet still hungry
- ☐ Crave sweets
- ☐ Crave Caffeine

(if more than hour after meal could be a crash from too much carb)

Approx. of macro Nutrient ratios of meal

% Carbs _____
% Protein _____
% Fat _____
Foods Eaten: _____
_____
_____
_____
_____
_____

MEAL 3 – TIME: _____

Most likely too many carbs

- ☐ Headache
- ☐ Anxiety
- ☐ Jittery/wired
- ☐ Difficulty concentrating
- ☐ Hunger is not satisfied
- ☐ Crave sweet
- ☐ Crave Protein & fat

Balanced Responses

- ☐ Appetite feels satisfied
- ☐ Feel emotionally balanced
- ☐ Good mental focus
- ☐ Normal level of energy
- ☐ No cravings for sweets
- ☐ No cravings for more food

Most likely too much protein &/or fat

- ☐ Lethargic
- ☐ Mentally Sluggish
- ☐ Heavy Gut
- ☐ Feel full yet still hungry
- ☐ Crave sweets
- ☐ Crave Caffeine

(if more than hour after meal could be a crash from too much carb)

Approx. of macro Nutrient ratios of meal

% Carbs _____
% Protein _____
% Fat _____
Foods Eaten: _____
_____
_____
_____
_____
_____

SNACKS:

Time: _____ Details: _____
Time: _____ Details: _____
Time: _____ Details: _____

DRINKS:

Details: _____
_____
_____

LIFESTYLE:

What time did you go to sleep? _____   What time did you get up? _____
Sleep quality? ☐ Sound ☐ Restless   Did you have night Sweats? ☐ Yes ☐ No
Did you awake during night (give time & reason)? _____
Did you wake up refreshed today or tired? ☐ Refreshed ☐ Tired
Did you start slow this morning? ☐ Yes ☐ No   If yes, how long did it take to feel alert? _____

Bowel movement(s)?
(number, colour, size & shape)
_____
_____

MOVEMENT :

Details: _____
_____
_____

GENERAL:

How did you feel today? _____
_____
_____

OTHER INFO: _____

219

DAILY FOOD & LIFESTYLE DIARY

DAILY FOOD DIARY - DATE: _____

MEAL 1 – TIME: _____

Complete everyday for 12 weeks

Please fill out form 1-2 hours after each meal

Most likely too many carbs
- ☐ Headache
- ☐ Anxiety
- ☐ Jittery/wired
- ☐ Difficulty concentrating
- ☐ Hunger is not satisfied
- ☐ Crave sweet
- ☐ Crave Protein & fat

Balanced Responses
- ☐ Appetite feels satisfied
- ☐ Feel emotionally balanced
- ☐ Good mental focus
- ☐ Normal level of energy
- ☐ No cravings for sweets
- ☐ No cravings for more food

Most likely too much protein &/or fat
- ☐ Lethargic
- ☐ Mentally Sluggish
- ☐ Heavy Gut
- ☐ Feel full yet still hungry
- ☐ Crave sweets
- ☐ Crave Caffeine
(if more than hour after meal could be a crash from too much carb)

Approx. of macro Nutrient ratios of meal
% Carbs _____
% Protein _____
% Fat _____
Foods Eaten: _____
_____
_____
_____
_____
_____

MEAL 2 – TIME: _____

Most likely too many carbs
- ☐ Headache
- ☐ Anxiety
- ☐ Jittery/wired
- ☐ Difficulty concentrating
- ☐ Hunger is not satisfied
- ☐ Crave sweet
- ☐ Crave Protein & fat

Balanced Responses
- ☐ Appetite feels satisfied
- ☐ Feel emotionally balanced
- ☐ Good mental focus
- ☐ Normal level of energy
- ☐ No cravings for sweets
- ☐ No cravings for more food

Most likely too much protein &/or fat
- ☐ Lethargic
- ☐ Mentally Sluggish
- ☐ Heavy Gut
- ☐ Feel full yet still hungry
- ☐ Crave sweets
- ☐ Crave Caffeine
(if more than hour after meal could be a crash from too much carb)

Approx. of macro Nutrient ratios of meal
% Carbs _____
% Protein _____
% Fat _____
Foods Eaten: _____
_____
_____
_____
_____
_____

MEAL 3 – TIME: _____

Most likely too many carbs
- ☐ Headache
- ☐ Anxiety
- ☐ Jittery/wired
- ☐ Difficulty concentrating
- ☐ Hunger is not satisfied
- ☐ Crave sweet
- ☐ Crave Protein & fat

Balanced Responses
- ☐ Appetite feels satisfied
- ☐ Feel emotionally balanced
- ☐ Good mental focus
- ☐ Normal level of energy
- ☐ No cravings for sweets
- ☐ No cravings for more food

Most likely too much protein &/or fat
- ☐ Lethargic
- ☐ Mentally Sluggish
- ☐ Heavy Gut
- ☐ Feel full yet still hungry
- ☐ Crave sweets
- ☐ Crave Caffeine
(if more than hour after meal could be a crash from too much carb)

Approx. of macro Nutrient ratios of meal
% Carbs _____
% Protein _____
% Fat _____
Foods Eaten: _____
_____
_____
_____
_____
_____

SNACKS:
Time: _____ Details: _____
Time: _____ Details: _____
Time: _____ Details: _____

DRINKS:
Details: _____
_____
_____

LIFESTYLE:
What time did you go to sleep? _____ What time did you get up? _____ Bowel movement(s)?
Sleep quality? ☐ Sound ☐ Restless   Did you have night Sweats? ☐ Yes ☐ No   (number, colour, size & shape)
Did you awake during night (give time & reason)? _____
Did you wake up refreshed today or tired? ☐ Refreshed ☐ Tired
Did you start slow this morning? ☐ Yes ☐ No   If yes, how long did it take to feel alert? _____

MOVEMENT :
Details: _____
_____
_____

GENERAL:
How did you feel today? _____
_____
_____

OTHER INFO: _____

DAILY FOOD & LIFESTYLE DIARY

DAILY FOOD DIARY - DATE: _____

Complete everyday for 12 weeks

MEAL 1 – TIME: _____

Please fill out form 1-2 hours after each meal

Most likely too many carbs	Balanced Responses	Most likely too much protein &/or fat	
☐ Headache	☐ Appetite feels satisfied	☐ Lethargic	Approx. of macro Nutrient ratios of meal
☐ Anxiety	☐ Feel emotionally balanced	☐ Mentally Sluggish	% Carbs _____
☐ Jittery/wired	☐ Good mental focus	☐ Heavy Gut	% Protein _____
☐ Difficulty concentrating	☐ Normal level of energy	☐ Feel full yet still hungry	% Fat _____
☐ Hunger is not satisfied	☐ No cravings for sweets	☐ Crave sweets	Foods Eaten: _____
☐ Crave sweet	☐ No cravings for more food	☐ Crave Caffeine	_____
☐ Crave Protein & fat		(if more than hour after meal could	_____
		be a crash from too much carb)	_____
			_____
			_____

MEAL 2 – TIME: _____

Most likely too many carbs	Balanced Responses	Most likely too much protein &/or fat	
☐ Headache	☐ Appetite feels satisfied	☐ Lethargic	Approx. of macro Nutrient ratios of meal
☐ Anxiety	☐ Feel emotionally balanced	☐ Mentally Sluggish	% Carbs _____
☐ Jittery/wired	☐ Good mental focus	☐ Heavy Gut	% Protein _____
☐ Difficulty concentrating	☐ Normal level of energy	☐ Feel full yet still hungry	% Fat _____
☐ Hunger is not satisfied	☐ No cravings for sweets	☐ Crave sweets	Foods Eaten: _____
☐ Crave sweet	☐ No cravings for more food	☐ Crave Caffeine	_____
☐ Crave Protein & fat		(if more than hour after meal could	_____
		be a crash from too much carb)	_____
			_____
			_____

MEAL 3 – TIME: _____

Most likely too many carbs	Balanced Responses	Most likely too much protein &/or fat	
☐ Headache	☐ Appetite feels satisfied	☐ Lethargic	Approx. of macro Nutrient ratios of meal
☐ Anxiety	☐ Feel emotionally balanced	☐ Mentally Sluggish	% Carbs _____
☐ Jittery/wired	☐ Good mental focus	☐ Heavy Gut	% Protein _____
☐ Difficulty concentrating	☐ Normal level of energy	☐ Feel full yet still hungry	% Fat _____
☐ Hunger is not satisfied	☐ No cravings for sweets	☐ Crave sweets	Foods Eaten: _____
☐ Crave sweet	☐ No cravings for more food	☐ Crave Caffeine	_____
☐ Crave Protein & fat		(if more than hour after meal could	_____
		be a crash from too much carb)	_____
			_____
			_____

SNACKS:

Time: _____ Details: _____

Time: _____ Details: _____

Time: _____ Details: _____

DRINKS:

Details: _____

_____

_____

LIFESTYLE:

What time did you go to sleep? _____ What time did you get up? _____ Bowel movement(s)?

Sleep quality? ☐ Sound ☐ Restless Did you have night Sweats? ☐ Yes ☐ No (number, colour, size & shape)

Did you awake during night (give time & reason)? _____ _____

Did you wake up refreshed today or tired? ☐ Refreshed ☐ Tired _____

Did you start slow this morning? ☐ Yes ☐ No If yes, how long did it take to feel alert? _____

MOVEMENT :

Details: _____

_____

GENERAL:

How did you feel today? _____

_____

OTHER INFO: _____

DAILY FOOD & LIFESTYLE DIARY

DAILY FOOD DIARY - DATE: _____   Complete everyday for 12 weeks

MEAL 1 – TIME: _____   Please fill out form 1-2 hours after each meal

Most likely too many carbs	Balanced Responses	Most likely too much protein &/or fat	
☐ Headache	☐ Appetite feels satisfied	☐ Lethargic	Approx. of macro Nutrient ratios of meal
☐ Anxiety	☐ Feel emotionally balanced	☐ Mentally Sluggish	% Carbs _____
☐ Jittery/wired	☐ Good mental focus	☐ Heavy Gut	% Protein _____
☐ Difficulty concentrating	☐ Normal level of energy	☐ Feel full yet still hungry	% Fat _____
☐ Hunger is not satisfied	☐ No cravings for sweets	☐ Crave sweets	Foods Eaten: _____
☐ Crave sweet	☐ No cravings for more food	☐ Crave Caffeine	_____
☐ Crave Protein & fat		(if more than hour after meal could	_____
		be a crash from too much carb)	_____
			_____
			_____

MEAL 2 – TIME: _____

Most likely too many carbs	Balanced Responses	Most likely too much protein &/or fat	
☐ Headache	☐ Appetite feels satisfied	☐ Lethargic	Approx. of macro Nutrient ratios of meal
☐ Anxiety	☐ Feel emotionally balanced	☐ Mentally Sluggish	% Carbs _____
☐ Jittery/wired	☐ Good mental focus	☐ Heavy Gut	% Protein _____
☐ Difficulty concentrating	☐ Normal level of energy	☐ Feel full yet still hungry	% Fat _____
☐ Hunger is not satisfied	☐ No cravings for sweets	☐ Crave sweets	Foods Eaten: _____
☐ Crave sweet	☐ No cravings for more food	☐ Crave Caffeine	_____
☐ Crave Protein & fat		(if more than hour after meal could	_____
		be a crash from too much carb)	_____
			_____
			_____

MEAL 3 – TIME: _____

Most likely too many carbs	Balanced Responses	Most likely too much protein &/or fat	
☐ Headache	☐ Appetite feels satisfied	☐ Lethargic	Approx. of macro Nutrient ratios of meal
☐ Anxiety	☐ Feel emotionally balanced	☐ Mentally Sluggish	% Carbs _____
☐ Jittery/wired	☐ Good mental focus	☐ Heavy Gut	% Protein _____
☐ Difficulty concentrating	☐ Normal level of energy	☐ Feel full yet still hungry	% Fat _____
☐ Hunger is not satisfied	☐ No cravings for sweets	☐ Crave sweets	Foods Eaten: _____
☐ Crave sweet	☐ No cravings for more food	☐ Crave Caffeine	_____
☐ Crave Protein & fat		(if more than hour after meal could	_____
		be a crash from too much carb)	_____
			_____
			_____

SNACKS: **DRINKS:**

Time: _____ Details: _____   Details: _____

Time: _____ Details: _____   _____

Time: _____ Details: _____   _____

LIFESTYLE:

What time did you go to sleep? _____   What time did you get up? _____   Bowel movement(s)?

Sleep quality? ☐ Sound ☐ Restless   Did you have night Sweats? ☐ Yes ☐ No   (number, colour, size & shape)

Did you awake during night (give time & reason)? _____   _____

Did you wake up refreshed today or tired? ☐ Refreshed ☐ Tired   _____

Did you start slow this morning? ☐ Yes ☐ No   If yes, how long did it take to feel alert? _____

MOVEMENT :   **GENERAL:**

Details: _____   How did you feel today? _____

_____   _____

_____   _____

OTHER INFO: _____

DAILY FOOD & LIFESTYLE DIARY

DAILY FOOD DIARY - DATE: _____

Complete everyday for 12 weeks

MEAL 1 – TIME: _____

Please fill out form 1-2 hours after each meal

Most likely too many carbs

- ☐ Headache
- ☐ Anxiety
- ☐ Jittery/wired
- ☐ Difficulty concentrating
- ☐ Hunger is not satisfied
- ☐ Crave sweet
- ☐ Crave Protein & fat

Balanced Responses

- ☐ Appetite feels satisfied
- ☐ Feel emotionally balanced
- ☐ Good mental focus
- ☐ Normal level of energy
- ☐ No cravings for sweets
- ☐ No cravings for more food

Most likely too much protein &/or fat

- ☐ Lethargic
- ☐ Mentally Sluggish
- ☐ Heavy Gut
- ☐ Feel full yet still hungry
- ☐ Crave sweets
- ☐ Crave Caffeine

(if more than hour after meal could be a crash from too much carb)

Approx. of macro Nutrient ratios of meal
% Carbs _____
% Protein _____
% Fat _____
Foods Eaten: _____
_____
_____
_____
_____
_____

MEAL 2 – TIME: _____

Most likely too many carbs

- ☐ Headache
- ☐ Anxiety
- ☐ Jittery/wired
- ☐ Difficulty concentrating
- ☐ Hunger is not satisfied
- ☐ Crave sweet
- ☐ Crave Protein & fat

Balanced Responses

- ☐ Appetite feels satisfied
- ☐ Feel emotionally balanced
- ☐ Good mental focus
- ☐ Normal level of energy
- ☐ No cravings for sweets
- ☐ No cravings for more food

Most likely too much protein &/or fat

- ☐ Lethargic
- ☐ Mentally Sluggish
- ☐ Heavy Gut
- ☐ Feel full yet still hungry
- ☐ Crave sweets
- ☐ Crave Caffeine

(if more than hour after meal could be a crash from too much carb)

Approx. of macro Nutrient ratios of meal
% Carbs _____
% Protein _____
% Fat _____
Foods Eaten: _____
_____
_____
_____
_____
_____

MEAL 3 – TIME: _____

Most likely too many carbs

- ☐ Headache
- ☐ Anxiety
- ☐ Jittery/wired
- ☐ Difficulty concentrating
- ☐ Hunger is not satisfied
- ☐ Crave sweet
- ☐ Crave Protein & fat

Balanced Responses

- ☐ Appetite feels satisfied
- ☐ Feel emotionally balanced
- ☐ Good mental focus
- ☐ Normal level of energy
- ☐ No cravings for sweets
- ☐ No cravings for more food

Most likely too much protein &/or fat

- ☐ Lethargic
- ☐ Mentally Sluggish
- ☐ Heavy Gut
- ☐ Feel full yet still hungry
- ☐ Crave sweets
- ☐ Crave Caffeine

(if more than hour after meal could be a crash from too much carb)

Approx. of macro Nutrient ratios of meal
% Carbs _____
% Protein _____
% Fat _____
Foods Eaten: _____
_____
_____
_____
_____
_____

SNACKS:

Time: _____ Details: _____
Time: _____ Details: _____
Time: _____ Details: _____

DRINKS:

Details: _____
_____
_____

LIFESTYLE:

What time did you go to sleep? _____ What time did you get up? _____
Sleep quality? ☐ Sound ☐ Restless   Did you have night Sweats? ☐ Yes ☐ No
Did you awake during night (give time & reason)? _____
Did you wake up refreshed today or tired? ☐ Refreshed ☐ Tired
Did you start slow this morning? ☐ Yes ☐ No   If yes, how long did it take to feel alert? _____

Bowel movement(s)?
(number, colour, size & shape)
_____
_____

MOVEMENT :

Details: _____
_____
_____

GENERAL:

How did you feel today? _____
_____
_____

OTHER INFO: _____

DAILY FOOD & LIFESTYLE DIARY

DAILY FOOD DIARY - DATE: _____

Complete everyday for 12 weeks

MEAL 1 – TIME: _____

Please fill out form 1-2 hours after each meal

Most likely too many carbs

- ☐ Headache
- ☐ Anxiety
- ☐ Jittery/wired
- ☐ Difficulty concentrating
- ☐ Hunger is not satisfied
- ☐ Crave sweet
- ☐ Crave Protein & fat

Balanced Responses

- ☐ Appetite feels satisfied
- ☐ Feel emotionally balanced
- ☐ Good mental focus
- ☐ Normal level of energy
- ☐ No cravings for sweets
- ☐ No cravings for more food

Most likely too much protein &/or fat

- ☐ Lethargic
- ☐ Mentally Sluggish
- ☐ Heavy Gut
- ☐ Feel full yet still hungry
- ☐ Crave sweets
- ☐ Crave Caffeine

(if more than hour after meal could be a crash from too much carb)

Approx. of macro Nutrient ratios of meal
% Carbs _____
% Protein _____
% Fat _____
Foods Eaten: _____
_____
_____
_____
_____
_____

MEAL 2 – TIME: _____

Most likely too many carbs

- ☐ Headache
- ☐ Anxiety
- ☐ Jittery/wired
- ☐ Difficulty concentrating
- ☐ Hunger is not satisfied
- ☐ Crave sweet
- ☐ Crave Protein & fat

Balanced Responses

- ☐ Appetite feels satisfied
- ☐ Feel emotionally balanced
- ☐ Good mental focus
- ☐ Normal level of energy
- ☐ No cravings for sweets
- ☐ No cravings for more food

Most likely too much protein &/or fat

- ☐ Lethargic
- ☐ Mentally Sluggish
- ☐ Heavy Gut
- ☐ Feel full yet still hungry
- ☐ Crave sweets
- ☐ Crave Caffeine

(if more than hour after meal could be a crash from too much carb)

Approx. of macro Nutrient ratios of meal
% Carbs _____
% Protein _____
% Fat _____
Foods Eaten: _____
_____
_____
_____
_____
_____

MEAL 3 – TIME: _____

Most likely too many carbs

- ☐ Headache
- ☐ Anxiety
- ☐ Jittery/wired
- ☐ Difficulty concentrating
- ☐ Hunger is not satisfied
- ☐ Crave sweet
- ☐ Crave Protein & fat

Balanced Responses

- ☐ Appetite feels satisfied
- ☐ Feel emotionally balanced
- ☐ Good mental focus
- ☐ Normal level of energy
- ☐ No cravings for sweets
- ☐ No cravings for more food

Most likely too much protein &/or fat

- ☐ Lethargic
- ☐ Mentally Sluggish
- ☐ Heavy Gut
- ☐ Feel full yet still hungry
- ☐ Crave sweets
- ☐ Crave Caffeine

(if more than hour after meal could be a crash from too much carb)

Approx. of macro Nutrient ratios of meal
% Carbs _____
% Protein _____
% Fat _____
Foods Eaten: _____
_____
_____
_____
_____
_____

SNACKS:

Time: _____ Details: _____
Time: _____ Details: _____
Time: _____ Details: _____

DRINKS:

Details: _____
_____
_____

LIFESTYLE:

What time did you go to sleep?_____ What time did you get up? _____ Bowel movement(s)?
Sleep quality? ☐ Sound ☐ Restless   Did you have night Sweats? ☐ Yes ☐ No   (number, colour, size & shape)
Did you awake during night (give time & reason)? _____
Did you wake up refreshed today or tired? ☐ Refreshed ☐ Tired   _____
Did you start slow this morning? ☐ Yes ☐ No   If yes, how long did it take to feel alert? _____

MOVEMENT :

Details: _____
_____
_____

GENERAL:

How did you feel today? _____
_____
_____

OTHER INFO: _____

DAILY FOOD & LIFESTYLE DIARY

DAILY FOOD DIARY - DATE: _____

Complete everyday for 12 weeks

MEAL 1 – TIME: _____

Please fill out form 1-2 hours after each meal

Most likely too many carbs

☐ Headache
☐ Anxiety
☐ Jittery/wired
☐ Difficulty concentrating
☐ Hunger is not satisfied
☐ Crave sweet
☐ Crave Protein & fat

Balanced Responses

☐ Appetite feels satisfied
☐ Feel emotionally balanced
☐ Good mental focus
☐ Normal level of energy
☐ No cravings for sweets
☐ No cravings for more food

Most likely too much protein &/or fat

☐ Lethargic
☐ Mentally Sluggish
☐ Heavy Gut
☐ Feel full yet still hungry
☐ Crave sweets
☐ Crave Caffeine
(if more than hour after meal could be a crash from too much carb)

Approx. of macro Nutrient ratios of meal
% Carbs _____
% Protein _____
% Fat _____
Foods Eaten: _____
_____
_____
_____
_____

MEAL 2 – TIME: _____

Most likely too many carbs

☐ Headache
☐ Anxiety
☐ Jittery/wired
☐ Difficulty concentrating
☐ Hunger is not satisfied
☐ Crave sweet
☐ Crave Protein & fat

Balanced Responses

☐ Appetite feels satisfied
☐ Feel emotionally balanced
☐ Good mental focus
☐ Normal level of energy
☐ No cravings for sweets
☐ No cravings for more food

Most likely too much protein &/or fat

☐ Lethargic
☐ Mentally Sluggish
☐ Heavy Gut
☐ Feel full yet still hungry
☐ Crave sweets
☐ Crave Caffeine
(if more than hour after meal could be a crash from too much carb)

Approx. of macro Nutrient ratios of meal
% Carbs _____
% Protein _____
% Fat _____
Foods Eaten: _____
_____
_____
_____
_____

MEAL 3 – TIME: _____

Most likely too many carbs

☐ Headache
☐ Anxiety
☐ Jittery/wired
☐ Difficulty concentrating
☐ Hunger is not satisfied
☐ Crave sweet
☐ Crave Protein & fat

Balanced Responses

☐ Appetite feels satisfied
☐ Feel emotionally balanced
☐ Good mental focus
☐ Normal level of energy
☐ No cravings for sweets
☐ No cravings for more food

Most likely too much protein &/or fat

☐ Lethargic
☐ Mentally Sluggish
☐ Heavy Gut
☐ Feel full yet still hungry
☐ Crave sweets
☐ Crave Caffeine
(if more than hour after meal could be a crash from too much carb)

Approx. of macro Nutrient ratios of meal
% Carbs _____
% Protein _____
% Fat _____
Foods Eaten: _____
_____
_____
_____
_____

SNACKS:

Time: _____ Details: _____
Time: _____ Details: _____
Time: _____ Details: _____

DRINKS:

Details: _____
_____
_____

LIFESTYLE:

What time did you go to sleep? _____   What time did you get up? _____
Sleep quality? ☐ Sound ☐ Restless   Did you have night Sweats? ☐ Yes ☐ No
Did you awake during night (give time & reason)? _____
Did you wake up refreshed today or tired? ☐ Refreshed ☐ Tired
Did you start slow this morning? ☐ Yes ☐ No   If yes, how long did it take to feel alert? _____

Bowel movement(s)?
(number, colour, size & shape)
_____
_____

MOVEMENT :

Details: _____
_____
_____

GENERAL:

How did you feel today? _____
_____
_____

OTHER INFO: _____

225

DAILY FOOD & LIFESTYLE DIARY

DAILY FOOD DIARY - DATE: _____

Complete everyday for 12 weeks

MEAL 1 – TIME: _____

Please fill out form 1-2 hours after each meal

Most likely too many carbs
- ☐ Headache
- ☐ Anxiety
- ☐ Jittery/wired
- ☐ Difficulty concentrating
- ☐ Hunger is not satisfied
- ☐ Crave sweet
- ☐ Crave Protein & fat

Balanced Responses
- ☐ Appetite feels satisfied
- ☐ Feel emotionally balanced
- ☐ Good mental focus
- ☐ Normal level of energy
- ☐ No cravings for sweets
- ☐ No cravings for more food

Most likely too much protein &/or fat
- ☐ Lethargic
- ☐ Mentally Sluggish
- ☐ Heavy Gut
- ☐ Feel full yet still hungry
- ☐ Crave sweets
- ☐ Crave Caffeine
(if more than hour after meal could be a crash from too much carb)

Approx. of macro Nutrient ratios of meal
% Carbs _____
% Protein _____
% Fat _____
Foods Eaten: _____
_____
_____
_____
_____
_____

MEAL 2 – TIME: _____

Most likely too many carbs
- ☐ Headache
- ☐ Anxiety
- ☐ Jittery/wired
- ☐ Difficulty concentrating
- ☐ Hunger is not satisfied
- ☐ Crave sweet
- ☐ Crave Protein & fat

Balanced Responses
- ☐ Appetite feels satisfied
- ☐ Feel emotionally balanced
- ☐ Good mental focus
- ☐ Normal level of energy
- ☐ No cravings for sweets
- ☐ No cravings for more food

Most likely too much protein &/or fat
- ☐ Lethargic
- ☐ Mentally Sluggish
- ☐ Heavy Gut
- ☐ Feel full yet still hungry
- ☐ Crave sweets
- ☐ Crave Caffeine
(if more than hour after meal could be a crash from too much carb)

Approx. of macro Nutrient ratios of meal
% Carbs _____
% Protein _____
% Fat _____
Foods Eaten: _____
_____
_____
_____
_____
_____

MEAL 3 – TIME: _____

Most likely too many carbs
- ☐ Headache
- ☐ Anxiety
- ☐ Jittery/wired
- ☐ Difficulty concentrating
- ☐ Hunger is not satisfied
- ☐ Crave sweet
- ☐ Crave Protein & fat

Balanced Responses
- ☐ Appetite feels satisfied
- ☐ Feel emotionally balanced
- ☐ Good mental focus
- ☐ Normal level of energy
- ☐ No cravings for sweets
- ☐ No cravings for more food

Most likely too much protein &/or fat
- ☐ Lethargic
- ☐ Mentally Sluggish
- ☐ Heavy Gut
- ☐ Feel full yet still hungry
- ☐ Crave sweets
- ☐ Crave Caffeine
(if more than hour after meal could be a crash from too much carb)

Approx. of macro Nutrient ratios of meal
% Carbs _____
% Protein _____
% Fat _____
Foods Eaten: _____
_____
_____
_____
_____
_____

SNACKS:
Time: _____ Details: _____
Time: _____ Details: _____
Time: _____ Details: _____

DRINKS:
Details: _____
_____
_____

LIFESTYLE:
What time did you go to sleep?_____ What time did you get up? _____
Sleep quality? ☐ Sound ☐ Restless   Did you have night Sweats? ☐ Yes ☐ No
Did you awake during night (give time & reason)? _____
Did you wake up refreshed today or tired? ☐ Refreshed ☐ Tired
Did you start slow this morning? ☐ Yes ☐ No   If yes, how long did it take to feel alert? _____

Bowel movement(s)?
(number, colour, size & shape)
_____
_____

MOVEMENT :
Details:_____
_____
_____

GENERAL:
How did you feel today? _____
_____
_____

OTHER INFO: _____

DAILY FOOD & LIFESTYLE DIARY

DAILY FOOD DIARY - DATE: _____

Complete everyday for 12 weeks

MEAL 1 – TIME: _____

Please fill out form 1-2 hours after each meal

Most likely too many carbs

- ☐ Headache
- ☐ Anxiety
- ☐ Jittery/wired
- ☐ Difficulty concentrating
- ☐ Hunger is not satisfied
- ☐ Crave sweet
- ☐ Crave Protein & fat

Balanced Responses

- ☐ Appetite feels satisfied
- ☐ Feel emotionally balanced
- ☐ Good mental focus
- ☐ Normal level of energy
- ☐ No cravings for sweets
- ☐ No cravings for more food

Most likely too much protein &/or fat

- ☐ Lethargic
- ☐ Mentally Sluggish
- ☐ Heavy Gut
- ☐ Feel full yet still hungry
- ☐ Crave sweets
- ☐ Crave Caffeine

(if more than hour after meal could be a crash from too much carb)

Approx. of macro Nutrient ratios of meal
% Carbs _____
% Protein _____
% Fat _____
Foods Eaten: _____
_____
_____
_____
_____
_____

MEAL 2 – TIME: _____

Most likely too many carbs

- ☐ Headache
- ☐ Anxiety
- ☐ Jittery/wired
- ☐ Difficulty concentrating
- ☐ Hunger is not satisfied
- ☐ Crave sweet
- ☐ Crave Protein & fat

Balanced Responses

- ☐ Appetite feels satisfied
- ☐ Feel emotionally balanced
- ☐ Good mental focus
- ☐ Normal level of energy
- ☐ No cravings for sweets
- ☐ No cravings for more food

Most likely too much protein &/or fat

- ☐ Lethargic
- ☐ Mentally Sluggish
- ☐ Heavy Gut
- ☐ Feel full yet still hungry
- ☐ Crave sweets
- ☐ Crave Caffeine

(if more than hour after meal could be a crash from too much carb)

Approx. of macro Nutrient ratios of meal
% Carbs _____
% Protein _____
% Fat _____
Foods Eaten: _____
_____
_____
_____
_____
_____

MEAL 3 – TIME: _____

Most likely too many carbs

- ☐ Headache
- ☐ Anxiety
- ☐ Jittery/wired
- ☐ Difficulty concentrating
- ☐ Hunger is not satisfied
- ☐ Crave sweet
- ☐ Crave Protein & fat

Balanced Responses

- ☐ Appetite feels satisfied
- ☐ Feel emotionally balanced
- ☐ Good mental focus
- ☐ Normal level of energy
- ☐ No cravings for sweets
- ☐ No cravings for more food

Most likely too much protein &/or fat

- ☐ Lethargic
- ☐ Mentally Sluggish
- ☐ Heavy Gut
- ☐ Feel full yet still hungry
- ☐ Crave sweets
- ☐ Crave Caffeine

(if more than hour after meal could be a crash from too much carb)

Approx. of macro Nutrient ratios of meal
% Carbs _____
% Protein _____
% Fat _____
Foods Eaten: _____
_____
_____
_____
_____

SNACKS:

Time: _____ Details: _____
Time: _____ Details: _____
Time: _____ Details: _____

DRINKS:

Details: _____
_____
_____

LIFESTYLE:

What time did you go to sleep?_____ What time did you get up? _____
Sleep quality? ☐ Sound ☐ Restless   Did you have night Sweats? ☐ Yes ☐ No
Did you awake during night (give time & reason)? _____
Did you wake up refreshed today or tired? ☐ Refreshed ☐ Tired
Did you start slow this morning? ☐ Yes ☐ No   If yes, how long did it take to feel alert? _____

Bowel movement(s)?
(number, colour, size & shape)
_____
_____

MOVEMENT :

Details: _____
_____
_____

GENERAL:

How did you feel today? _____
_____
_____

OTHER INFO: _____

DAILY FOOD & LIFESTYLE DIARY

DAILY FOOD DIARY - DATE: _____

Complete everyday for 12 weeks

MEAL 1 – TIME: _____

Please fill out form 1-2 hours after each meal

Most likely too many carbs

☐ Headache
☐ Anxiety
☐ Jittery/wired
☐ Difficulty concentrating
☐ Hunger is not satisfied
☐ Crave sweet
☐ Crave Protein & fat

Balanced Responses

☐ Appetite feels satisfied
☐ Feel emotionally balanced
☐ Good mental focus
☐ Normal level of energy
☐ No cravings for sweets
☐ No cravings for more food

Most likely too much protein &/or fat

☐ Lethargic
☐ Mentally Sluggish
☐ Heavy Gut
☐ Feel full yet still hungry
☐ Crave sweets
☐ Crave Caffeine
(if more than hour after meal could be a crash from too much carb)

Approx. of macro Nutrient ratios of meal
% Carbs _____
% Protein _____
% Fat _____
Foods Eaten: _____
_____
_____
_____
_____
_____

MEAL 2 – TIME: _____

Most likely too many carbs

☐ Headache
☐ Anxiety
☐ Jittery/wired
☐ Difficulty concentrating
☐ Hunger is not satisfied
☐ Crave sweet
☐ Crave Protein & fat

Balanced Responses

☐ Appetite feels satisfied
☐ Feel emotionally balanced
☐ Good mental focus
☐ Normal level of energy
☐ No cravings for sweets
☐ No cravings for more food

Most likely too much protein &/or fat

☐ Lethargic
☐ Mentally Sluggish
☐ Heavy Gut
☐ Feel full yet still hungry
☐ Crave sweets
☐ Crave Caffeine
(if more than hour after meal could be a crash from too much carb)

Approx. of macro Nutrient ratios of meal
% Carbs _____
% Protein _____
% Fat _____
Foods Eaten: _____
_____
_____
_____
_____
_____

MEAL 3 – TIME: _____

Most likely too many carbs

☐ Headache
☐ Anxiety
☐ Jittery/wired
☐ Difficulty concentrating
☐ Hunger is not satisfied
☐ Crave sweet
☐ Crave Protein & fat

Balanced Responses

☐ Appetite feels satisfied
☐ Feel emotionally balanced
☐ Good mental focus
☐ Normal level of energy
☐ No cravings for sweets
☐ No cravings for more food

Most likely too much protein &/or fat

☐ Lethargic
☐ Mentally Sluggish
☐ Heavy Gut
☐ Feel full yet still hungry
☐ Crave sweets
☐ Crave Caffeine
(if more than hour after meal could be a crash from too much carb)

Approx. of macro Nutrient ratios of meal
% Carbs _____
% Protein _____
% Fat _____
Foods Eaten: _____
_____
_____
_____
_____
_____

SNACKS:

Time: _____ Details: _____
Time: _____ Details: _____
Time: _____ Details: _____

DRINKS:

Details: _____
_____
_____

LIFESTYLE:

What time did you go to sleep? _____ What time did you get up? _____ Bowel movement(s)?
Sleep quality? ☐ Sound ☐ Restless Did you have night Sweats? ☐ Yes ☐ No (number, colour, size & shape)
Did you awake during night (give time & reason)? _____
Did you wake up refreshed today or tired? ☐ Refreshed ☐ Tired
Did you start slow this morning? ☐ Yes ☐ No If yes, how long did it take to feel alert? _____

MOVEMENT :

Details: _____
_____
_____

GENERAL:

How did you feel today? _____
_____
_____

OTHER INFO: _____

DAILY FOOD & LIFESTYLE DIARY

DAILY FOOD DIARY - DATE: _____

Complete everyday for 12 weeks

MEAL 1 – TIME: _____

Please fill out form 1-2 hours after each meal

Most likely too many carbs

- ☐ Headache
- ☐ Anxiety
- ☐ Jittery/wired
- ☐ Difficulty concentrating
- ☐ Hunger is not satisfied
- ☐ Crave sweet
- ☐ Crave Protein & fat

Balanced Responses

- ☐ Appetite feels satisfied
- ☐ Feel emotionally balanced
- ☐ Good mental focus
- ☐ Normal level of energy
- ☐ No cravings for sweets
- ☐ No cravings for more food

Most likely too much protein &/or fat

- ☐ Lethargic
- ☐ Mentally Sluggish
- ☐ Heavy Gut
- ☐ Feel full yet still hungry
- ☐ Crave sweets
- ☐ Crave Caffeine

(if more than hour after meal could be a crash from too much carb)

Approx. of macro Nutrient ratios of meal
% Carbs _____
% Protein _____
% Fat _____
Foods Eaten: _____
_____
_____
_____
_____
_____

MEAL 2 – TIME: _____

Most likely too many carbs

- ☐ Headache
- ☐ Anxiety
- ☐ Jittery/wired
- ☐ Difficulty concentrating
- ☐ Hunger is not satisfied
- ☐ Crave sweet
- ☐ Crave Protein & fat

Balanced Responses

- ☐ Appetite feels satisfied
- ☐ Feel emotionally balanced
- ☐ Good mental focus
- ☐ Normal level of energy
- ☐ No cravings for sweets
- ☐ No cravings for more food

Most likely too much protein &/or fat

- ☐ Lethargic
- ☐ Mentally Sluggish
- ☐ Heavy Gut
- ☐ Feel full yet still hungry
- ☐ Crave sweets
- ☐ Crave Caffeine

(if more than hour after meal could be a crash from too much carb)

Approx. of macro Nutrient ratios of meal
% Carbs _____
% Protein _____
% Fat _____
Foods Eaten: _____
_____
_____
_____
_____
_____

MEAL 3 – TIME: _____

Most likely too many carbs

- ☐ Headache
- ☐ Anxiety
- ☐ Jittery/wired
- ☐ Difficulty concentrating
- ☐ Hunger is not satisfied
- ☐ Crave sweet
- ☐ Crave Protein & fat

Balanced Responses

- ☐ Appetite feels satisfied
- ☐ Feel emotionally balanced
- ☐ Good mental focus
- ☐ Normal level of energy
- ☐ No cravings for sweets
- ☐ No cravings for more food

Most likely too much protein &/or fat

- ☐ Lethargic
- ☐ Mentally Sluggish
- ☐ Heavy Gut
- ☐ Feel full yet still hungry
- ☐ Crave sweets
- ☐ Crave Caffeine

(if more than hour after meal could be a crash from too much carb)

Approx. of macro Nutrient ratios of meal
% Carbs _____
% Protein _____
% Fat _____
Foods Eaten: _____
_____
_____
_____
_____
_____

SNACKS:

Time: _____ Details: _____
Time: _____ Details: _____
Time: _____ Details: _____

DRINKS:

Details: _____
_____
_____

LIFESTYLE:

What time did you go to sleep? _____ What time did you get up? _____
Sleep quality? ☐ Sound ☐ Restless   Did you have night Sweats? ☐ Yes ☐ No
Did you awake during night (give time & reason)? _____
Did you wake up refreshed today or tired? ☐ Refreshed ☐ Tired
Did you start slow this morning? ☐ Yes ☐ No   If yes, how long did it take to feel alert? _____

Bowel movement(s)?
(number, colour, size & shape)
_____
_____

MOVEMENT :

Details: _____
_____
_____

GENERAL:

How did you feel today? _____
_____
_____

OTHER INFO: _____

DAILY FOOD & LIFESTYLE DIARY

DAILY FOOD DIARY - DATE: _____

Complete everyday for 12 weeks

MEAL 1 – TIME: _____

Please fill out form 1-2 hours after each meal

Most likely too many carbs
- [ ] Headache
- [ ] Anxiety
- [ ] Jittery/wired
- [ ] Difficulty concentrating
- [ ] Hunger is not satisfied
- [ ] Crave sweet
- [ ] Crave Protein & fat

Balanced Responses
- [ ] Appetite feels satisfied
- [ ] Feel emotionally balanced
- [ ] Good mental focus
- [ ] Normal level of energy
- [ ] No cravings for sweets
- [ ] No cravings for more food

Most likely too much protein &/or fat
- [ ] Lethargic
- [ ] Mentally Sluggish
- [ ] Heavy Gut
- [ ] Feel full yet still hungry
- [ ] Crave sweets
- [ ] Crave Caffeine

(if more than hour after meal could be a crash from too much carb)

Approx. of macro Nutrient ratios of meal
% Carbs _____
% Protein _____
% Fat _____
Foods Eaten: _____
_____
_____
_____
_____
_____

MEAL 2 – TIME: _____

Most likely too many carbs
- [ ] Headache
- [ ] Anxiety
- [ ] Jittery/wired
- [ ] Difficulty concentrating
- [ ] Hunger is not satisfied
- [ ] Crave sweet
- [ ] Crave Protein & fat

Balanced Responses
- [ ] Appetite feels satisfied
- [ ] Feel emotionally balanced
- [ ] Good mental focus
- [ ] Normal level of energy
- [ ] No cravings for sweets
- [ ] No cravings for more food

Most likely too much protein &/or fat
- [ ] Lethargic
- [ ] Mentally Sluggish
- [ ] Heavy Gut
- [ ] Feel full yet still hungry
- [ ] Crave sweets
- [ ] Crave Caffeine

(if more than hour after meal could be a crash from too much carb)

Approx. of macro Nutrient ratios of meal
% Carbs _____
% Protein _____
% Fat _____
Foods Eaten: _____
_____
_____
_____
_____

MEAL 3 – TIME: _____

Most likely too many carbs
- [ ] Headache
- [ ] Anxiety
- [ ] Jittery/wired
- [ ] Difficulty concentrating
- [ ] Hunger is not satisfied
- [ ] Crave sweet
- [ ] Crave Protein & fat

Balanced Responses
- [ ] Appetite feels satisfied
- [ ] Feel emotionally balanced
- [ ] Good mental focus
- [ ] Normal level of energy
- [ ] No cravings for sweets
- [ ] No cravings for more food

Most likely too much protein &/or fat
- [ ] Lethargic
- [ ] Mentally Sluggish
- [ ] Heavy Gut
- [ ] Feel full yet still hungry
- [ ] Crave sweets
- [ ] Crave Caffeine

(if more than hour after meal could be a crash from too much carb)

Approx. of macro Nutrient ratios of meal
% Carbs _____
% Protein _____
% Fat _____
Foods Eaten: _____
_____
_____
_____
_____

SNACKS:
Time: _____ Details: _____
Time: _____ Details: _____
Time: _____ Details: _____

DRINKS:
Details: _____
_____
_____

LIFESTYLE:
What time did you go to sleep? _____   What time did you get up? _____
Sleep quality? [ ] Sound [ ] Restless   Did you have night Sweats? [ ] Yes [ ] No
Did you awake during night (give time & reason)? _____
Did you wake up refreshed today or tired? [ ] Refreshed [ ] Tired
Did you start slow this morning? [ ] Yes [ ] No   If yes, how long did it take to feel alert? _____

Bowel movement(s)?
(number, colour, size & shape)
_____
_____

MOVEMENT :
Details: _____
_____
_____

GENERAL:
How did you feel today? _____
_____
_____

OTHER INFO: _____

DAILY FOOD & LIFESTYLE DIARY

DAILY FOOD DIARY - DATE: _____

Complete everyday for 12 weeks

MEAL 1 – TIME: _____

Please fill out form 1-2 hours after each meal

Most likely too many carbs	Balanced Responses	Most likely too much protein &/or fat	
☐ Headache	☐ Appetite feels satisfied	☐ Lethargic	Approx. of macro Nutrient ratios of meal
☐ Anxiety	☐ Feel emotionally balanced	☐ Mentally Sluggish	% Carbs _____
☐ Jittery/wired	☐ Good mental focus	☐ Heavy Gut	% Protein _____
☐ Difficulty concentrating	☐ Normal level of energy	☐ Feel full yet still hungry	% Fat _____
☐ Hunger is not satisfied	☐ No cravings for sweets	☐ Crave sweets	Foods Eaten: _____
☐ Crave sweet	☐ No cravings for more food	☐ Crave Caffeine	_____
☐ Crave Protein & fat		(if more than hour after meal could	_____
		be a crash from too much carb)	_____
			_____
			_____

MEAL 2 – TIME: _____

Most likely too many carbs	Balanced Responses	Most likely too much protein &/or fat	
☐ Headache	☐ Appetite feels satisfied	☐ Lethargic	Approx. of macro Nutrient ratios of meal
☐ Anxiety	☐ Feel emotionally balanced	☐ Mentally Sluggish	% Carbs _____
☐ Jittery/wired	☐ Good mental focus	☐ Heavy Gut	% Protein _____
☐ Difficulty concentrating	☐ Normal level of energy	☐ Feel full yet still hungry	% Fat _____
☐ Hunger is not satisfied	☐ No cravings for sweets	☐ Crave sweets	Foods Eaten: _____
☐ Crave sweet	☐ No cravings for more food	☐ Crave Caffeine	_____
☐ Crave Protein & fat		(if more than hour after meal could	_____
		be a crash from too much carb)	_____
			_____
			_____

MEAL 3 – TIME: _____

Most likely too many carbs	Balanced Responses	Most likely too much protein &/or fat	
☐ Headache	☐ Appetite feels satisfied	☐ Lethargic	Approx. of macro Nutrient ratios of meal
☐ Anxiety	☐ Feel emotionally balanced	☐ Mentally Sluggish	% Carbs _____
☐ Jittery/wired	☐ Good mental focus	☐ Heavy Gut	% Protein _____
☐ Difficulty concentrating	☐ Normal level of energy	☐ Feel full yet still hungry	% Fat _____
☐ Hunger is not satisfied	☐ No cravings for sweets	☐ Crave sweets	Foods Eaten: _____
☐ Crave sweet	☐ No cravings for more food	☐ Crave Caffeine	_____
☐ Crave Protein & fat		(if more than hour after meal could	_____
		he a crash from too much carb)	_____
			_____

SNACKS:

Time: _____ Details: _____
Time: _____ Details: _____
Time: _____ Details: _____

DRINKS:

Details: _____
_____
_____

LIFESTYLE:

What time did you go to sleep? _____   What time did you get up? _____
Sleep quality? ☐ Sound ☐ Restless   Did you have night Sweats? ☐ Yes ☐ No
Did you awake during night (give time & reason)? _____
Did you wake up refreshed today or tired? ☐ Refreshed ☐ Tired
Did you start slow this morning? ☐ Yes ☐ No   If yes, how long did it take to feel alert? _____

Bowel movement(s)?
(number, colour, size & shape)

_____
_____

MOVEMENT :

Details: _____
_____
_____

GENERAL:

How did you feel today? _____
_____
_____

OTHER INFO: _____

231

DAILY FOOD & LIFESTYLE DIARY

DAILY FOOD DIARY - DATE: _____

Complete everyday for 12 weeks

Please fill out form 1-2 hours after each meal

MEAL 1 – TIME: _____

Most likely too many carbs

- ☐ Headache
- ☐ Anxiety
- ☐ Jittery/wired
- ☐ Difficulty concentrating
- ☐ Hunger is not satisfied
- ☐ Crave sweet
- ☐ Crave Protein & fat

Balanced Responses

- ☐ Appetite feels satisfied
- ☐ Feel emotionally balanced
- ☐ Good mental focus
- ☐ Normal level of energy
- ☐ No cravings for sweets
- ☐ No cravings for more food

Most likely too much protein &/or fat

- ☐ Lethargic
- ☐ Mentally Sluggish
- ☐ Heavy Gut
- ☐ Feel full yet still hungry
- ☐ Crave sweets
- ☐ Crave Caffeine

(if more than hour after meal could be a crash from too much carb)

Approx. of macro Nutrient ratios of meal

% Carbs _____
% Protein _____
% Fat _____
Foods Eaten: _____
_____
_____
_____
_____
_____

MEAL 2 – TIME: _____

Most likely too many carbs

- ☐ Headache
- ☐ Anxiety
- ☐ Jittery/wired
- ☐ Difficulty concentrating
- ☐ Hunger is not satisfied
- ☐ Crave sweet
- ☐ Crave Protein & fat

Balanced Responses

- ☐ Appetite feels satisfied
- ☐ Feel emotionally balanced
- ☐ Good mental focus
- ☐ Normal level of energy
- ☐ No cravings for sweets
- ☐ No cravings for more food

Most likely too much protein &/or fat

- ☐ Lethargic
- ☐ Mentally Sluggish
- ☐ Heavy Gut
- ☐ Feel full yet still hungry
- ☐ Crave sweets
- ☐ Crave Caffeine

(if more than hour after meal could be a crash from too much carb)

Approx. of macro Nutrient ratios of meal

% Carbs _____
% Protein _____
% Fat _____
Foods Eaten: _____
_____
_____
_____
_____
_____

MEAL 3 – TIME: _____

Most likely too many carbs

- ☐ Headache
- ☐ Anxiety
- ☐ Jittery/wired
- ☐ Difficulty concentrating
- ☐ Hunger is not satisfied
- ☐ Crave sweet
- ☐ Crave Protein & fat

Balanced Responses

- ☐ Appetite feels satisfied
- ☐ Feel emotionally balanced
- ☐ Good mental focus
- ☐ Normal level of energy
- ☐ No cravings for sweets
- ☐ No cravings for more food

Most likely too much protein &/or fat

- ☐ Lethargic
- ☐ Mentally Sluggish
- ☐ Heavy Gut
- ☐ Feel full yet still hungry
- ☐ Crave sweets
- ☐ Crave Caffeine

(if more than hour after meal could be a crash from too much carb)

Approx. of macro Nutrient ratios of meal

% Carbs _____
% Protein _____
% Fat _____
Foods Eaten: _____
_____
_____
_____
_____
_____

SNACKS:

Time: _____ Details: _____
Time: _____ Details: _____
Time: _____ Details: _____

DRINKS:

Details: _____
_____
_____

LIFESTYLE:

What time did you go to sleep? _____ What time did you get up? _____
Sleep quality? ☐ Sound ☐ Restless   Did you have night Sweats? ☐ Yes ☐ No
Did you awake during night (give time & reason)? _____
Did you wake up refreshed today or tired? ☐ Refreshed ☐ Tired
Did you start slow this morning? ☐ Yes ☐ No   If yes, how long did it take to feel alert? _____

Bowel movement(s)?
(number, colour, size & shape)
_____
_____

MOVEMENT :

Details: _____
_____
_____

GENERAL:

How did you feel today? _____
_____
_____

OTHER INFO: _____

DAILY FOOD & LIFESTYLE DIARY

DAILY FOOD DIARY - DATE: _____

MEAL 1 – TIME: _____

Complete everyday for 12 weeks

Please fill out form 1-2 hours after each meal

Most likely too many carbs	Balanced Responses	Most likely too much protein &/or fat	
☐ Headache	☐ Appetite feels satisfied	☐ Lethargic	Approx. of macro Nutrient ratios of meal
☐ Anxiety	☐ Feel emotionally balanced	☐ Mentally Sluggish	% Carbs _____
☐ Jittery/wired	☐ Good mental focus	☐ Heavy Gut	% Protein _____
☐ Difficulty concentrating	☐ Normal level of energy	☐ Feel full yet still hungry	% Fat _____
☐ Hunger is not satisfied	☐ No cravings for sweets	☐ Crave sweets	Foods Eaten: _____
☐ Crave sweet	☐ No cravings for more food	☐ Crave Caffeine	_____
☐ Crave Protein & fat		(if more than hour after meal could be a crash from too much carb)	_____ _____ _____ _____

MEAL 2 – TIME: _____

Most likely too many carbs	Balanced Responses	Most likely too much protein &/or fat	
☐ Headache	☐ Appetite feels satisfied	☐ Lethargic	Approx. of macro Nutrient ratios of meal
☐ Anxiety	☐ Feel emotionally balanced	☐ Mentally Sluggish	% Carbs _____
☐ Jittery/wired	☐ Good mental focus	☐ Heavy Gut	% Protein _____
☐ Difficulty concentrating	☐ Normal level of energy	☐ Feel full yet still hungry	% Fat _____
☐ Hunger is not satisfied	☐ No cravings for sweets	☐ Crave sweets	Foods Eaten: _____
☐ Crave sweet	☐ No cravings for more food	☐ Crave Caffeine	_____
☐ Crave Protein & fat		(if more than hour after meal could be a crash from too much carb)	_____ _____ _____ _____

MEAL 3 – TIME: _____

Most likely too many carbs	Balanced Responses	Most likely too much protein &/or fat	
☐ Headache	☐ Appetite feels satisfied	☐ Lethargic	Approx. of macro Nutrient ratios of meal
☐ Anxiety	☐ Feel emotionally balanced	☐ Mentally Sluggish	% Carbs _____
☐ Jittery/wired	☐ Good mental focus	☐ Heavy Gut	% Protein _____
☐ Difficulty concentrating	☐ Normal level of energy	☐ Feel full yet still hungry	% Fat _____
☐ Hunger is not satisfied	☐ No cravings for sweets	☐ Crave sweets	Foods Eaten: _____
☐ Crave sweet	☐ No cravings for more food	☐ Crave Caffeine	_____
☐ Crave Protein & fat		(if more than hour after meal could be a crash from too much carb)	_____ _____ _____ _____

SNACKS:

Time: _____ Details: _____

Time: _____ Details: _____

Time: _____ Details: _____

DRINKS:

Details: _____

_____

_____

LIFESTYLE:

What time did you go to sleep?_____ What time did you get up? _____

Sleep quality? ☐ Sound ☐ Restless Did you have night Sweats? ☐ Yes ☐ No

Did you awake during night (give time & reason)? _____

Did you wake up refreshed today or tired? ☐ Refreshed ☐ Tired

Did you start slow this morning? ☐ Yes ☐ No If yes, how long did it take to feel alert? _____

Bowel movement(s)?
(number, colour, size & shape)

_____

_____

MOVEMENT :

Details: _____

_____

GENERAL:

How did you feel today? _____

_____

OTHER INFO: _____

DAILY FOOD & LIFESTYLE DIARY

DAILY FOOD DIARY - DATE: _____

Complete everyday for 12 weeks

MEAL 1 – TIME: _____

Please fill out form 1-2 hours after each meal

Most likely too many carbs	Balanced Responses	Most likely too much protein &/or fat	
☐ Headache	☐ Appetite feels satisfied	☐ Lethargic	Approx. of macro Nutrient ratios of meal
☐ Anxiety	☐ Feel emotionally balanced	☐ Mentally Sluggish	% Carbs _____
☐ Jittery/wired	☐ Good mental focus	☐ Heavy Gut	% Protein _____
☐ Difficulty concentrating	☐ Normal level of energy	☐ Feel full yet still hungry	% Fat _____
☐ Hunger is not satisfied	☐ No cravings for sweets	☐ Crave sweets	Foods Eaten: _____
☐ Crave sweet	☐ No cravings for more food	☐ Crave Caffeine	_____
☐ Crave Protein & fat		(if more than hour after meal could	_____
		be a crash from too much carb)	_____

MEAL 2 – TIME: _____

Most likely too many carbs	Balanced Responses	Most likely too much protein &/or fat	
☐ Headache	☐ Appetite feels satisfied	☐ Lethargic	Approx. of macro Nutrient ratios of meal
☐ Anxiety	☐ Feel emotionally balanced	☐ Mentally Sluggish	% Carbs _____
☐ Jittery/wired	☐ Good mental focus	☐ Heavy Gut	% Protein _____
☐ Difficulty concentrating	☐ Normal level of energy	☐ Feel full yet still hungry	% Fat _____
☐ Hunger is not satisfied	☐ No cravings for sweets	☐ Crave sweets	Foods Eaten: _____
☐ Crave sweet	☐ No cravings for more food	☐ Crave Caffeine	_____
☐ Crave Protein & fat		(if more than hour after meal could	_____
		be a crash from too much carb)	_____

MEAL 3 – TIME: _____

Most likely too many carbs	Balanced Responses	Most likely too much protein &/or fat	
☐ Headache	☐ Appetite feels satisfied	☐ Lethargic	Approx. of macro Nutrient ratios of meal
☐ Anxiety	☐ Feel emotionally balanced	☐ Mentally Sluggish	% Carbs _____
☐ Jittery/wired	☐ Good mental focus	☐ Heavy Gut	% Protein _____
☐ Difficulty concentrating	☐ Normal level of energy	☐ Feel full yet still hungry	% Fat _____
☐ Hunger is not satisfied	☐ No cravings for sweets	☐ Crave sweets	Foods Eaten: _____
☐ Crave sweet	☐ No cravings for more food	☐ Crave Caffeine	_____
☐ Crave Protein & fat		(if more than hour after meal could	_____
		be a crash from too much carb)	_____

SNACKS:

Time: _____ Details: _____
Time: _____ Details: _____
Time: _____ Details: _____

DRINKS:

Details: _____
_____
_____

LIFESTYLE:

What time did you go to sleep? _____ What time did you get up? _____
Sleep quality? ☐ Sound ☐ Restless   Did you have night Sweats? ☐ Yes ☐ No
Did you awake during night (give time & reason)? _____
Did you wake up refreshed today or tired? ☐ Refreshed ☐ Tired
Did you start slow this morning? ☐ Yes ☐ No   If yes, how long did it take to feel alert? _____

Bowel movement(s)?
(number, colour, size & shape)
_____
_____

MOVEMENT :

Details: _____
_____
_____

GENERAL:

How did you feel today? _____
_____
_____

OTHER INFO: _____

DAILY FOOD & LIFESTYLE DIARY

DAILY FOOD DIARY - DATE: _____

Complete everyday for 12 weeks

Please fill out form 1-2 hours after each meal

MEAL 1 – TIME: _____

Most likely too many carbs

- ☐ Headache
- ☐ Anxiety
- ☐ Jittery/wired
- ☐ Difficulty concentrating
- ☐ Hunger is not satisfied
- ☐ Crave sweet
- ☐ Crave Protein & fat

Balanced Responses

- ☐ Appetite feels satisfied
- ☐ Feel emotionally balanced
- ☐ Good mental focus
- ☐ Normal level of energy
- ☐ No cravings for sweets
- ☐ No cravings for more food

Most likely too much protein &/or fat

- ☐ Lethargic
- ☐ Mentally Sluggish
- ☐ Heavy Gut
- ☐ Feel full yet still hungry
- ☐ Crave sweets
- ☐ Crave Caffeine

(if more than hour after meal could be a crash from too much carb)

Approx. of macro Nutrient ratios of meal
% Carbs _____
% Protein _____
% Fat _____
Foods Eaten: _____
_____
_____
_____
_____
_____

MEAL 2 – TIME: _____

Most likely too many carbs

- ☐ Headache
- ☐ Anxiety
- ☐ Jittery/wired
- ☐ Difficulty concentrating
- ☐ Hunger is not satisfied
- ☐ Crave sweet
- ☐ Crave Protein & fat

Balanced Responses

- ☐ Appetite feels satisfied
- ☐ Feel emotionally balanced
- ☐ Good mental focus
- ☐ Normal level of energy
- ☐ No cravings for sweets
- ☐ No cravings for more food

Most likely too much protein &/or fat

- ☐ Lethargic
- ☐ Mentally Sluggish
- ☐ Heavy Gut
- ☐ Feel full yet still hungry
- ☐ Crave sweets
- ☐ Crave Caffeine

(if more than hour after meal could be a crash from too much carb)

Approx. of macro Nutrient ratios of meal
% Carbs _____
% Protein _____
% Fat _____
Foods Eaten: _____
_____
_____
_____
_____
_____

MEAL 3 – TIME: _____

Most likely too many carbs

- ☐ Headache
- ☐ Anxiety
- ☐ Jittery/wired
- ☐ Difficulty concentrating
- ☐ Hunger is not satisfied
- ☐ Crave sweet
- ☐ Crave Protein & fat

Balanced Responses

- ☐ Appetite feels satisfied
- ☐ Feel emotionally balanced
- ☐ Good mental focus
- ☐ Normal level of energy
- ☐ No cravings for sweets
- ☐ No cravings for more food

Most likely too much protein &/or fat

- ☐ Lethargic
- ☐ Mentally Sluggish
- ☐ Heavy Gut
- ☐ Feel full yet still hungry
- ☐ Crave sweets
- ☐ Crave Caffeine

(if more than hour after meal could be a crash from too much carb)

Approx. of macro Nutrient ratios of meal
% Carbs _____
% Protein _____
% Fat _____
Foods Eaten: _____
_____
_____
_____
_____

SNACKS:

Time: _____ Details: _____
Time: _____ Details: _____
Time: _____ Details: _____

DRINKS:

Details: _____
_____
_____

LIFESTYLE:

What time did you go to sleep? _____   What time did you get up? _____
Sleep quality? ☐ Sound ☐ Restless   Did you have night Sweats? ☐ Yes ☐ No
Did you awake during night (give time & reason)? _____
Did you wake up refreshed today or tired? ☐ Refreshed ☐ Tired
Did you start slow this morning? ☐ Yes ☐ No   If yes, how long did it take to feel alert? _____

Bowel movement(s)?
(number, colour, size & shape)
_____
_____

MOVEMENT :

Details: _____
_____
_____

GENERAL:

How did you feel today? _____
_____
_____

OTHER INFO: _____

DAILY FOOD & LIFESTYLE DIARY

DAILY FOOD DIARY - DATE: _____

Complete everyday for 12 weeks

MEAL 1 – TIME: _____

Please fill out form 1-2 hours after each meal

Most likely too many carbs

- ☐ Headache
- ☐ Anxiety
- ☐ Jittery/wired
- ☐ Difficulty concentrating
- ☐ Hunger is not satisfied
- ☐ Crave sweet
- ☐ Crave Protein & fat

Balanced Responses

- ☐ Appetite feels satisfied
- ☐ Feel emotionally balanced
- ☐ Good mental focus
- ☐ Normal level of energy
- ☐ No cravings for sweets
- ☐ No cravings for more food

Most likely too much protein &/or fat

- ☐ Lethargic
- ☐ Mentally Sluggish
- ☐ Heavy Gut
- ☐ Feel full yet still hungry
- ☐ Crave sweets
- ☐ Crave Caffeine

(if more than hour after meal could be a crash from too much carb)

Approx. of macro Nutrient ratios of meal

% Carbs _____
% Protein _____
% Fat _____
Foods Eaten: _____
_____
_____
_____
_____
_____

MEAL 2 – TIME: _____

Most likely too many carbs

- ☐ Headache
- ☐ Anxiety
- ☐ Jittery/wired
- ☐ Difficulty concentrating
- ☐ Hunger is not satisfied
- ☐ Crave sweet
- ☐ Crave Protein & fat

Balanced Responses

- ☐ Appetite feels satisfied
- ☐ Feel emotionally balanced
- ☐ Good mental focus
- ☐ Normal level of energy
- ☐ No cravings for sweets
- ☐ No cravings for more food

Most likely too much protein &/or fat

- ☐ Lethargic
- ☐ Mentally Sluggish
- ☐ Heavy Gut
- ☐ Feel full yet still hungry
- ☐ Crave sweets
- ☐ Crave Caffeine

(if more than hour after meal could be a crash from too much carb)

Approx. of macro Nutrient ratios of meal

% Carbs _____
% Protein _____
% Fat _____
Foods Eaten: _____
_____
_____
_____
_____
_____

MEAL 3 – TIME: _____

Most likely too many carbs

- ☐ Headache
- ☐ Anxiety
- ☐ Jittery/wired
- ☐ Difficulty concentrating
- ☐ Hunger is not satisfied
- ☐ Crave sweet
- ☐ Crave Protein & fat

Balanced Responses

- ☐ Appetite feels satisfied
- ☐ Feel emotionally balanced
- ☐ Good mental focus
- ☐ Normal level of energy
- ☐ No cravings for sweets
- ☐ No cravings for more food

Most likely too much protein &/or fat

- ☐ Lethargic
- ☐ Mentally Sluggish
- ☐ Heavy Gut
- ☐ Feel full yet still hungry
- ☐ Crave sweets
- ☐ Crave Caffeine

(if more than hour after meal could be a crash from too much carb)

Approx. of macro Nutrient ratios of meal

% Carbs _____
% Protein _____
% Fat _____
Foods Eaten: _____
_____
_____
_____
_____
_____

SNACKS:

Time: _____ Details: _____
Time: _____ Details: _____
Time: _____ Details: _____

DRINKS:

Details: _____
_____
_____

LIFESTYLE:

What time did you go to sleep? _____ What time did you get up? _____ Bowel movement(s)?
Sleep quality? ☐ Sound ☐ Restless Did you have night Sweats? ☐ Yes ☐ No (number, colour, size & shape)
Did you awake during night (give time & reason)? _____
Did you wake up refreshed today or tired? ☐ Refreshed ☐ Tired
Did you start slow this morning? ☐ Yes ☐ No If yes, how long did it take to feel alert? _____

MOVEMENT :

Details: _____
_____
_____

GENERAL:

How did you feel today? _____
_____
_____

OTHER INFO: _____

DAILY FOOD & LIFESTYLE DIARY

DAILY FOOD DIARY - DATE: _____

Complete everyday for 12 weeks

Please fill out form 1-2 hours after each meal

MEAL 1 – TIME: _____

Most likely too many carbs

- ☐ Headache
- ☐ Anxiety
- ☐ Jittery/wired
- ☐ Difficulty concentrating
- ☐ Hunger is not satisfied
- ☐ Crave sweet
- ☐ Crave Protein & fat

Balanced Responses

- ☐ Appetite feels satisfied
- ☐ Feel emotionally balanced
- ☐ Good mental focus
- ☐ Normal level of energy
- ☐ No cravings for sweets
- ☐ No cravings for more food

Most likely too much protein &/or fat

- ☐ Lethargic
- ☐ Mentally Sluggish
- ☐ Heavy Gut
- ☐ Feel full yet still hungry
- ☐ Crave sweets
- ☐ Crave Caffeine

(if more than hour after meal could be a crash from too much carb)

Approx. of macro Nutrient ratios of meal
% Carbs _____
% Protein _____
% Fat _____
Foods Eaten: _____
_____
_____
_____
_____
_____

MEAL 2 – TIME: _____

Most likely too many carbs

- ☐ Headache
- ☐ Anxiety
- ☐ Jittery/wired
- ☐ Difficulty concentrating
- ☐ Hunger is not satisfied
- ☐ Crave sweet
- ☐ Crave Protein & fat

Balanced Responses

- ☐ Appetite feels satisfied
- ☐ Feel emotionally balanced
- ☐ Good mental focus
- ☐ Normal level of energy
- ☐ No cravings for sweets
- ☐ No cravings for more food

Most likely too much protein &/or fat

- ☐ Lethargic
- ☐ Mentally Sluggish
- ☐ Heavy Gut
- ☐ Feel full yet still hungry
- ☐ Crave sweets
- ☐ Crave Caffeine

(if more than hour after meal could be a crash from too much carb)

Approx. of macro Nutrient ratios of meal
% Carbs _____
% Protein _____
% Fat _____
Foods Eaten: _____
_____
_____
_____
_____

MEAL 3 – TIME: _____

Most likely too many carbs

- ☐ Headache
- ☐ Anxiety
- ☐ Jittery/wired
- ☐ Difficulty concentrating
- ☐ Hunger is not satisfied
- ☐ Crave sweet
- ☐ Crave Protein & fat

Balanced Responses

- ☐ Appetite feels satisfied
- ☐ Feel emotionally balanced
- ☐ Good mental focus
- ☐ Normal level of energy
- ☐ No cravings for sweets
- ☐ No cravings for more food

Most likely too much protein &/or fat

- ☐ Lethargic
- ☐ Mentally Sluggish
- ☐ Heavy Gut
- ☐ Feel full yet still hungry
- ☐ Crave sweets
- ☐ Crave Caffeine

(if more than hour after meal could be a crash from too much carb)

Approx. of macro Nutrient ratios of meal
% Carbs _____
% Protein _____
% Fat _____
Foods Eaten: _____
_____
_____
_____
_____

SNACKS:

Time: _____ Details: _____
Time: _____ Details: _____
Time: _____ Details: _____

DRINKS:

Details: _____
_____
_____

LIFESTYLE:

What time did you go to sleep? _____ What time did you get up? _____
Sleep quality? ☐ Sound ☐ Restless Did you have night Sweats? ☐ Yes ☐ No
Did you awake during night (give time & reason)? _____
Did you wake up refreshed today or tired? ☐ Refreshed ☐ Tired
Did you start slow this morning? ☐ Yes ☐ No   If yes, how long did it take to feel alert? _____

Bowel movement(s)?
(number, colour, size & shape)
_____
_____

MOVEMENT :

Details: _____
_____
_____

GENERAL:

How did you feel today? _____
_____
_____

OTHER INFO: _____

DAILY FOOD & LIFESTYLE DIARY

DAILY FOOD DIARY - DATE: _____

Complete everyday for 12 weeks

MEAL 1 – TIME: _____

Please fill out form 1-2 hours after each meal

Most likely too many carbs
- ☐ Headache
- ☐ Anxiety
- ☐ Jittery/wired
- ☐ Difficulty concentrating
- ☐ Hunger is not satisfied
- ☐ Crave sweet
- ☐ Crave Protein & fat

Balanced Responses
- ☐ Appetite feels satisfied
- ☐ Feel emotionally balanced
- ☐ Good mental focus
- ☐ Normal level of energy
- ☐ No cravings for sweets
- ☐ No cravings for more food

Most likely too much protein &/or fat
- ☐ Lethargic
- ☐ Mentally Sluggish
- ☐ Heavy Gut
- ☐ Feel full yet still hungry
- ☐ Crave sweets
- ☐ Crave Caffeine
(if more than hour after meal could be a crash from too much carb)

Approx. of macro Nutrient ratios of meal
% Carbs _____
% Protein _____
% Fat _____
Foods Eaten: _____
_____
_____
_____
_____
_____

MEAL 2 – TIME: _____

Most likely too many carbs
- ☐ Headache
- ☐ Anxiety
- ☐ Jittery/wired
- ☐ Difficulty concentrating
- ☐ Hunger is not satisfied
- ☐ Crave sweet
- ☐ Crave Protein & fat

Balanced Responses
- ☐ Appetite feels satisfied
- ☐ Feel emotionally balanced
- ☐ Good mental focus
- ☐ Normal level of energy
- ☐ No cravings for sweets
- ☐ No cravings for more food

Most likely too much protein &/or fat
- ☐ Lethargic
- ☐ Mentally Sluggish
- ☐ Heavy Gut
- ☐ Feel full yet still hungry
- ☐ Crave sweets
- ☐ Crave Caffeine
(if more than hour after meal could be a crash from too much carb)

Approx. of macro Nutrient ratios of meal
% Carbs _____
% Protein _____
% Fat _____
Foods Eaten: _____
_____
_____
_____
_____
_____

MEAL 3 – TIME: _____

Most likely too many carbs
- ☐ Headache
- ☐ Anxiety
- ☐ Jittery/wired
- ☐ Difficulty concentrating
- ☐ Hunger is not satisfied
- ☐ Crave sweet
- ☐ Crave Protein & fat

Balanced Responses
- ☐ Appetite feels satisfied
- ☐ Feel emotionally balanced
- ☐ Good mental focus
- ☐ Normal level of energy
- ☐ No cravings for sweets
- ☐ No cravings for more food

Most likely too much protein &/or fat
- ☐ Lethargic
- ☐ Mentally Sluggish
- ☐ Heavy Gut
- ☐ Feel full yet still hungry
- ☐ Crave sweets
- ☐ Crave Caffeine
(if more than hour after meal could be a crash from too much carb)

Approx. of macro Nutrient ratios of meal
% Carbs _____
% Protein _____
% Fat _____
Foods Eaten: _____
_____
_____
_____
_____
_____

SNACKS:

Time: _____ Details: _____
Time: _____ Details: _____
Time: _____ Details: _____

DRINKS:

Details: _____
_____
_____

LIFESTYLE:

What time did you go to sleep? _____ What time did you get up? _____
Sleep quality? ☐ Sound ☐ Restless   Did you have night Sweats? ☐ Yes ☐ No
Did you awake during night (give time & reason)? _____
Did you wake up refreshed today or tired? ☐ Refreshed ☐ Tired
Did you start slow this morning? ☐ Yes ☐ No   If yes, how long did it take to feel alert? _____

Bowel movement(s)?
(number, colour, size & shape)
_____
_____

MOVEMENT :

Details: _____
_____
_____

GENERAL:

How did you feel today? _____
_____
_____

OTHER INFO: _____

DAILY FOOD & LIFESTYLE DIARY

DAILY FOOD DIARY - DATE: _____

Complete everyday for 12 weeks

Please fill out form 1-2 hours after each meal

MEAL 1 – TIME: _____

Most likely too many carbs

- ☐ Headache
- ☐ Anxiety
- ☐ Jittery/wired
- ☐ Difficulty concentrating
- ☐ Hunger is not satisfied
- ☐ Crave sweet
- ☐ Crave Protein & fat

Balanced Responses

- ☐ Appetite feels satisfied
- ☐ Feel emotionally balanced
- ☐ Good mental focus
- ☐ Normal level of energy
- ☐ No cravings for sweets
- ☐ No cravings for more food

Most likely too much protein &/or fat

- ☐ Lethargic
- ☐ Mentally Sluggish
- ☐ Heavy Gut
- ☐ Feel full yet still hungry
- ☐ Crave sweets
- ☐ Crave Caffeine

(if more than hour after meal could be a crash from too much carb)

Approx. of macro Nutrient ratios of meal

% Carbs _____
% Protein _____
% Fat _____

Foods Eaten: _____
_____
_____
_____
_____
_____

MEAL 2 – TIME: _____

Most likely too many carbs

- ☐ Headache
- ☐ Anxiety
- ☐ Jittery/wired
- ☐ Difficulty concentrating
- ☐ Hunger is not satisfied
- ☐ Crave sweet
- ☐ Crave Protein & fat

Balanced Responses

- ☐ Appetite feels satisfied
- ☐ Feel emotionally balanced
- ☐ Good mental focus
- ☐ Normal level of energy
- ☐ No cravings for sweets
- ☐ No cravings for more food

Most likely too much protein &/or fat

- ☐ Lethargic
- ☐ Mentally Sluggish
- ☐ Heavy Gut
- ☐ Feel full yet still hungry
- ☐ Crave sweets
- ☐ Crave Caffeine

(if more than hour after meal could be a crash from too much carb)

Approx. of macro Nutrient ratios of meal

% Carbs _____
% Protein _____
% Fat _____

Foods Eaten: _____
_____
_____
_____
_____
_____

MEAL 3 – TIME: _____

Most likely too many carbs

- ☐ Headache
- ☐ Anxiety
- ☐ Jittery/wired
- ☐ Difficulty concentrating
- ☐ Hunger is not satisfied
- ☐ Crave sweet
- ☐ Crave Protein & fat

Balanced Responses

- ☐ Appetite feels satisfied
- ☐ Feel emotionally balanced
- ☐ Good mental focus
- ☐ Normal level of energy
- ☐ No cravings for sweets
- ☐ No cravings for more food

Most likely too much protein &/or fat

- ☐ Lethargic
- ☐ Mentally Sluggish
- ☐ Heavy Gut
- ☐ Feel full yet still hungry
- ☐ Crave sweets
- ☐ Crave Caffeine

(if more than hour after meal could be a crash from too much carb)

Approx. of macro Nutrient ratios of meal

% Carbs _____
% Protein _____
% Fat _____

Foods Eaten: _____
_____
_____
_____
_____
_____

SNACKS:

Time: _____ Details: _____
Time: _____ Details: _____
Time: _____ Details: _____

DRINKS:

Details: _____
_____
_____

LIFESTYLE:

What time did you go to sleep? _____ What time did you get up? _____

Sleep quality? ☐ Sound ☐ Restless   Did you have night Sweats? ☐ Yes ☐ No

Did you awake during night (give time & reason)? _____

Did you wake up refreshed today or tired? ☐ Refreshed ☐ Tired

Did you start slow this morning? ☐ Yes ☐ No   If yes, how long did it take to feel alert? _____

Bowel movement(s)?
(number, colour, size & shape)
_____
_____

MOVEMENT :

Details: _____
_____
_____

GENERAL:

How did you feel today? _____
_____
_____

OTHER INFO: _____

APPENDIX V
REFERENCES

American College of Sports Medicine, 'Health Fitness Instructor', 1998

Brown, S. 'Play', (2009) Penguin

Chek, P. 'How to Eat Move & Be Healthy' (2004) C.H.E.K. Institute

Chek, P. 'Last 4 Doctors You'll Ever Need' (2007) E-book C.H.E.K. Institute

Chek, P. 'Under the Veil of Deception' (2002) C.H.E.K. Institute

C.H.E.K. Institute, 'Practitioner & Holistic Lifestyle Coach Course notes'

Dalai Lama, 'The Art of Happiness' (1998) Coronet Books

Ding, J. '15 Minute Tai Chi' (2003) Thorsons

Douillard, J. 'Mind Body Sport' (2001) Three Rivers Press

Dreyer, D. 'Chi Running' (2003) Pocket Books

Dunbar, R. 'The Human Story' (2004) Faber and Faber

Dweck, C. 'Mindset' (2012) Robinson

Ecologist Online, 'The Big Fat Fix' (01.11.06)

Environment California Research and Policy Centre, 'Growing Up Toxic – Chemical Exposures and Increases in Developmental Disease' (June 2004)

Elkind, D. 'The Power of Play' (2007) Da Capo Lifelong Books

Fallon, S. 'Nourishing Traditions' (2001) New Trends

Forencich, F. 'Change Your Body, Change the World' (2010)

Forencich, F. 'Exuberant Animal' (2006)

Forencich, F. 'Exuberant Animal Play Book' (2009)

Forencich, F. 'Play as if your life depends on It' (2003)

Gill, T. 'No Fear - Growing Up in Risk Averse Society' (2007) Calouste Gulbenkian Foundation

Glasser, W. 'Choice Theory' (1998) Harper Perennial

Gluckman, P. & Hanson, M. 'Mismatch' (2006) Oxford University Press

Iacoboni, M. 'Mirroring People' (2008) Picador

James, O. 'Affluenza' (2007) Vermilion

Kendrick, M. 'The Great Cholesterol Con' (2008) John Blake Publishing

Kumar, S. 'Earth Pilgrim' (2009) Green Books

Lipton, B. 'Biology of Belief' (2005) Mountain of Love

Lipton, B. 'Spontaneous Evolution' (2010) Hay House

Louv, R. 'Last Child in the Woods' (2005) Atlantic Books

McDougall, C. 'Born to Run' (2009) Profile Books

McTaggert, L. 'What Doctors Don't Tell You' (2005) Thorsons

Neil, M. 'Super Coach' (2009) Hay House

Organic & Natural Living, extracts from Dr Paula Baillie-Hamilton book, 'The Detox Diet – Eliminate Chemicals Calories and Enhance Your Natural Slimming System" (Newsletter Issue 2)

Pert, C. 'Molecules of Emotion' (1997) Pocket Books

Rogers, S. 'Detoxify or Die' (2002) Sand Key Company

Rosenberg, M. 'Nonviolent Communication' (2003) Puddle Dancer

Ruiz, D. M. *'The Mastery of Love'* (1999) Amber-Allen

Sapolsky, R. *'Junk Food Monkeys'* (1997) Headline

Sapolsky, R. *'Why Zebras Don't Get Ulcers'* (2004) Owl Books

Schlosser, E. *'Fast Food Nation'* (2002)

Syed, M. *'Bounce'* (2010) Fourth Estate

The Happy Budda, *'Happiness & How It Happens'* (2011) Leaping Hare Press

Tolle, E. *'The Power of Now'* (2005) Hodder & Stoughton

Wallden, M. *'Barefoot Running Efficiency Research'* www.primallifestyle.com

Wiley, T.S. *'Lights Out'* (2000) Pocket Books

Williams, R. *'Biochemical Indviduality'* (1956) Keats Publishing

Wilson, J. *'Adrenal Fatigue'* (2002) Smart Publications

Winston, R. *'Human Instinct'* (2002) Bantam Books

Wolcott, W. & Fahey, T. *'The Metabolic Typing Diet'* (2000) Broadway Books

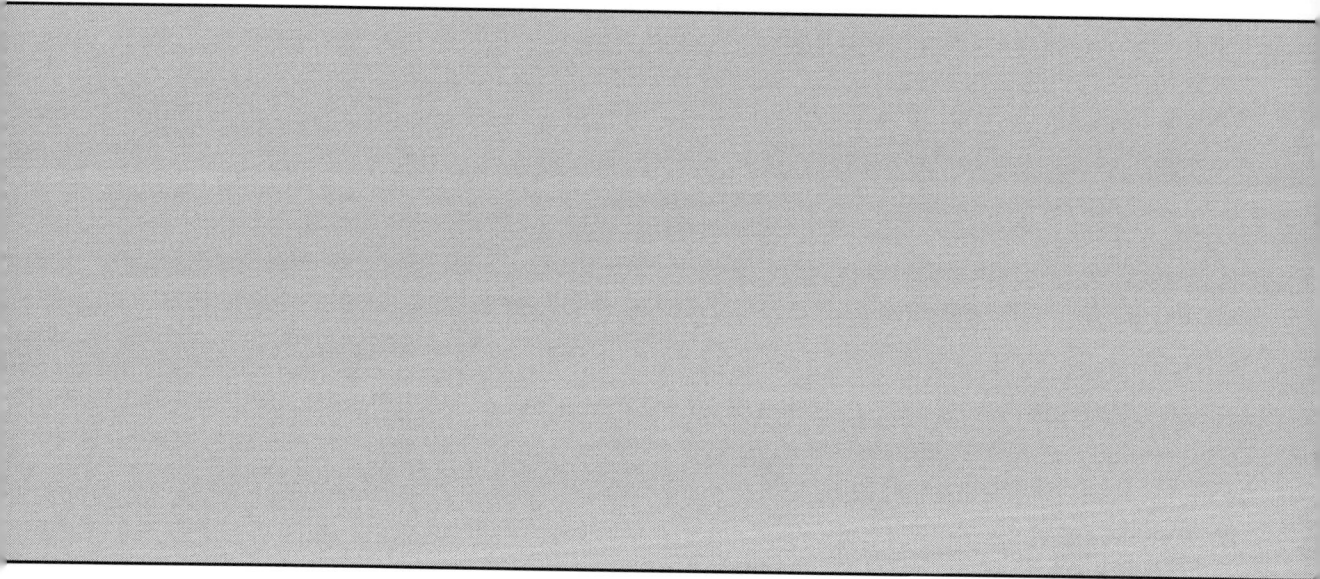

APPENDIC VI
FURTHER ACTIONS /
HELP

PRIVATE COACHING

HEALTH RETREATS

GROUP PRESENTATIONS

HEARTCHECK

Using the latest medical science of heart rate variability analysis this is a non-intrusive test to give you an exact and reproducible measure of your health.

ADVANCED METABOLIC TYPING™ ASSESSMENT

A detailed and personalised report to give you a starting point for understanding your body's unique biochemistry and for building a personalised diet for yourself.

HAIR MINERAL ANALYSIS

Gives a detailed report on your toxic load profile and mineral deficiency/balance.

C.H.E.K. BIOMECHANICAL ASSESSMENTS

Including posture, flexibility, core strength, movement screening, physiological load & corrective exercise programming.

BAREFOOT RUNNING COACHING

Visit www.takeshapehealth.co.uk for more information.

THANKYOU

Thank you to some inspirational teachers over years including clients, authors, educators, friends and family.

The amazing 'health' educators and authors include Frank Forencich aka 'The Exuberant Animal', Paul Chek, Emma Lane, Matthew Wallden, 'Barefoot Ted' McDonald and Dr Michael Kucera.

Thank you to my family, young and old, that have helped educate me either directly or indirectly!

Thank you for the help of my editors/proofreaders Nick Thomas and Susie Taylor. And lastly, thank you to Beth Snowden from The Write Factor for transforming the text into this wonderful book.

ABOUT THE AUTHOR

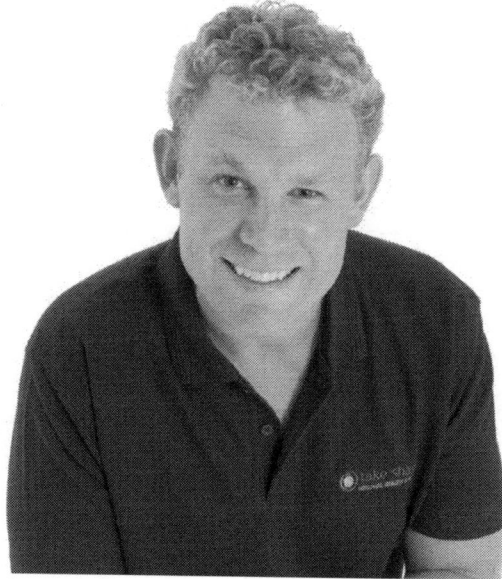

Ollie Martin has 20 years personal training experience and is one of the most qualified personal trainers in the country. He is a former semi-pro rugby player and is a sports scientist, a CHEK Practitioner and Holistic Lifestyle Coach. He runs his own health & performance company in Surrey, UK.

Ollie has consulted for a wide range of private clients, companies and sports teams. He has worked behind a desk, has a young family, runs a small business and so knows about time, family and work pressures. All his programmes take individuals and their pressures into account.

He can help anyone, any group or team improve their performance whether it is at work, sport or family time, if they choose to do so.

www.takeshapehealth.co.uk

"OLLIE HAS HELPED ME TO INCREASE MY ENERGY LEVELS AND GIVE ME A MUCH MORE POSITIVE OUTLOOK ON LIFE IN GENERAL."

PARTNER, EC HARRIS

"THE SEMINAR PROGRAMME WAS VERY INFORMATIVE, GAVE PLENTY OF FOOD FOR THOUGHT AND WERE VERY ENJOYABLE."

HM REVENUE & CUSTOMS

THE SEMINARS WERE FUN, INFORMATIVE & THOUGHT PROVOKING. THE MOVEMENT SESSIONS WERE INSPIRATIONAL & VERY MOTIVATING. THE PRESENTER WAS FRIENDLY & EASY GOING WITH LOTS OF DIFFERENT IDEAS OF HOW TO GET YOU MOVING & SHAKING."

THE WI, DENMAN COLLEGE

"OLLIE HAS BEEN A KEY MEMBER OF OUR TEAM AND HAS BEEN VERY PATIENT WITH US. HIS TAILOR-MADE TRAINING PROGRAMME NOT ONLY PREPARED ME FOR THE RACE, IT CHANGED MY LIFESTYLE FOR THE BETTER. I HAVE LOST LOADS OF WEIGHT AND FEEL GREAT AS A RESULT OF HIS TRAINING, AND I DON'T INTEND TO GO BACK TO THE WAY I WAS BEFORE."

SURREY MIRROR

"THANK YOU FOR HELPING THE NATION GET FITTER"

FIA COMMIT TO GET FIT

Made in the USA
Charleston, SC
20 August 2014